the
3a.m.
HANDBOOK

the
3a.m.
HANDBOOK

The Most Commonly Asked Questions
About Your Child's Health

EDITED BY WILLIAM FELDMAN, MD

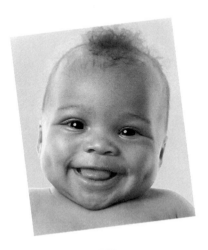

Facts On File, Inc.

The 3 a.m. Handbook

Facts On File, Inc.
11 Penn Plaza
New York, NY 10001

Library of Congress Cataloging-in-Publication Data

Feldman, William, M.D.
     The 3 a.m. handbook : the most commonly asked questions about your child's health / edited by William Feldman.
        p. cm.
     "First published in 1997 by Key Porter Books, Toronto, Ontario, Canada"—t.p. verso.
     ISBN 0-8160-3802-3
     1. Children—Health and hygiene—Miscellanea. 2. Infants—Health and hygiene—Miscellanea. 3. Pediatrics—Popular works.   I. Title. RJ61.F364   1997
618.92—dc21   97-52235

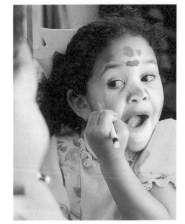

Editing: Gena Gorrell
Design: Leah Gryfe
Illustrations: John Lightfoot
Electronic formatting: Heidi Palfrey

Printed and bound in Canada

10 9 8 7 6 5 4 3 2 1

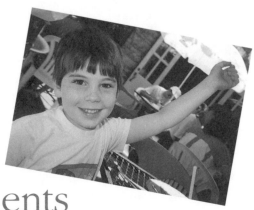

Acknowledgments

We wish to acknowledge Christabel Braganza, Administrative Assistant at the Hospital for Sick Children, for her hard work, organizational skills, and unflagging sense of humor. In addition, we are grateful to our editor, Gena Gorrell, and Claudia Anderson, Director of Public Affairs at the hospital, without whom this book would not have happened.

Acknowledgment of Photo Sources *Page 3*: Penny Gentieu/Tony Stone Images; *4*: Kevin Horan/Tony Stone Images; *6*: Lawrence Monneret/Tony Stone Images; *7, right*: Peter Correz/Tony Stone Images; *9, right*: David Stewart/Tony Stone Images; *11, right*: Andy Sacks/Tony Stone Images; *left*: Bruce Ayres/Tony Stone Images; *17, left*: Penny Gentieu/Tony Stone Images; *24, right*: Chronis Jons/Tony Stone Images; *left*: Steven Peters/Tony Stone Images; *39, right*: Penny Gentieu/Tony Stone Images; *left*: Andy Cox/Tony Stone Images; *50, left*: Richard Meats/Tony Stone Images; *57, right*: Joe McBride/Tony Stone Images; *70, right*: Penny Gentieu/Tony Stone Images; *left*: Tony Stone Images; *79*: Tamara Reynolds/Tony Stone Images; *87, right*: John Fortunato/Tony Stone Images; *97, right*: Peter Cade/Tony Stone Images; *left*: Nicole Katano/Tony Stone Images; *106*: Steven Peters/Tony Stone Images; *115, right*: Chad Slattery/Tony Stone Images; *132, right*: David Young Wolff/Tony Stone Images; *149, right*: David Harry Stewart/Tony Stone Images; *164, right*: Joe Cornish/Tony Stone Images; *left*: Jonathon Selig/Tony Stone Images; *187, left*: Peter Dazeley/Tony Stone Images; *198, right*: David Young Wolff/Tony Stone Images; *left*: Charles Thatcher/Tony Stone Images; *204, right*: Jurgen Reisch/Tony Stone Images; *left*: Walter Hodges/Tony Stone Images; *211*: Nicole Katano/Tony Stone Images.

Special Thanks to: *Page 5*: Matthew Thompson; *7*: Samuel Berson-Weinberg; *9, left*: Victor Copetti; *17, right*: Liam Kavanagh; *50, right*: Matthew and Roisín Thompson; *57, left*: Matthew Thompson; *87, left*: Scott Peters; *115, left*: Ryan Prendergast; *132, left*: Ben and Scott Peters; *149, left*: Liam Kavanagh; *187, right*: Leah Berson-Weinberg; *214*: Liam Kavanagh.

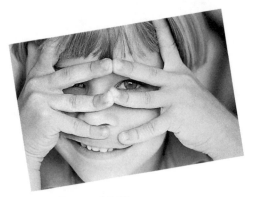

General Editor

William Feldman, MD, FRCPC

Coauthors

Paul Dick, MD, CM, FRCPC

Darcy Fehlings, MD, FRCPC

William Feldman, MD, FRCPC

Marvin Gans, MD, FRCPC

Alan Goldbloom, MD, FRCPC

Saul Greenberg, MD, FRCPC

William Hanley, MD, FRCPC

Robert Hilliard, MD, FRCPC

Moshe Ipp, MBBCh, FRCPC

Sheila Jacobson, MBBCh, FRCPC

David Lloyd, MD, FRCPC

Patricia Parkin, MD, FRCPC

Norman Saunders, MD, FRCPC

Clive Schwartz, MBBCh, FRCPC

Susan Tallett, MBBS, FRCPC

Lionel Weinstein, MD, FRCPC

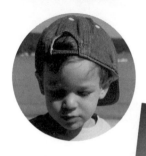

Contents

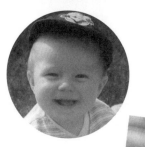

Introduction

· ·

The purpose of this book is to provide parents with general information about their children's health, based not just on opinion but on sound scientific evidence. No attempt has been made here to describe every disease and condition that can affect children; instead, this book covers extensively the troublesome aspects of "normal" behaviors of children, such as eating and sleeping problems.

All parents ask themselves "how" questions—"How can I protect my child from injuries?"; "How can I tell if there's something seriously wrong with my child?"; "How can I improve my child's eating habits?" For answers they often turn to their family doctors or pediatricians, or to books and articles by physicians. They look for answers that are based on years of practical experience.

Although the knowledge gained from practical experience is immensely valuable, it's not the only source—or necessarily the best one—for answers to those "how" questions. A doctor's conclusions may be affected by the particular population of patients he or she serves, or by his or her own philosophy or expectations. This "personal" aspect is the reason that hospitals and other medical institutions carry out a broad range of clinical research studies and controlled trials. By eliminating personal bias, and methodically comparing results in large numbers of children, it's possible to say with much more certainty what behavior is "normal" and what is not, what treatment "works" and what does not.

The authors of this book are all highly trained pediatricians, and members of the Division of General Pediatrics at the Hospital for Sick Children, in Toronto. All of us are also members—full-time or part-time—of the Department of Pediatrics at the University of Toronto. We all share a profound interest in "evidence-based medicine," medicine based on the science of clinical epidemiology—in other words, based on organized, disciplined research into how children really behave, how we can keep them healthy, and how we can best help them when they are unwell.

Collectively, of course, we have hundreds of years of personal experience in taking care of children, both healthy and sick. But while we are focusing on our individual child patients, we are also asking ourselves more general questions—the same "how" questions that parents ask—and looking for ways to test procedures and beliefs.

We hope the answers we've found will resolve some of the questions you've been asking yourselves, and will help you through the exciting, exhilarating, and sometimes *exasperating* challenge of raising your children to be the best they can be!

CHAPTER 1

Choosing Your Child's Doctor

• •

hen young doctors are about to go into practice, they often ask older physicians what they need to do to be successful. For many years the standard answer has been: "Demonstrate the three A's." They are, in order of importance, *ability*, *availability*, and *affability*. When you're choosing a doctor for your child, these are three essential qualities to keep in mind.

What exactly do you mean by "ability"?

In *Webster's New World Dictionary*, "ability" is defined as "power to do [something]; talent; skill." The powers, talents, and skills your child's doctor should have can be categorized into four broad areas: prevention, diagnosis, treatment, and rehabilitation.

In the field of *prevention*, your child's doctor should be aware of which preventive measures work and which don't. For example, certain screening tests for newborns are very effective in preventing mental or physical disability, and should be performed on all newborns. "Well-baby visits"—routine medical checkups when nothing seems to be wrong—provide immunization and advice that can prevent life-threatening problems later on.

Diagnosis means discovering the root of a problem such as fever, pain, difficult breathing, or disturbing behavior. The physician should be skilled at reaching a diagnosis by various means. The first and most important is simply asking the parents (and children, if they are not too young) for a description of the problem: whether it's getting better or worse, what makes it better or worse, how it's affecting the child's (and family's) life. The answers often go a long way towards identifying the cause of the problem. The second means of diagnosis is the physical examination. The third is laboratory tests. In general, the more experienced physicians are in diagnosing and treating the medical problems of children, the less they depend on lab tests. There are, of course, problems that require certain tests or X rays, but the most able diagnosticians rely heavily on asking questions and on physical exams.

The fourth means of diagnosis is referring the child to another doctor for consultation. Some doctors are so busy seeing large numbers of patients that they don't have time to ask the extra questions or to do the detailed physical examination needed for a diagnosis; they tend to refer too many children to consultants. Other doctors are overly confident of their own abilities, and they may not refer enough children to consultants.

Modern *treatment* has changed dramatically in the last hundred years. In the old days doctors didn't have a lot of effective medications or surgical procedures to offer, so they were much better at diagnosis than at treatment. In the last century, however, we have developed a host of effective treatments, as well as more sophisticated diagnostic tools. However, just as the treatments have become more powerful, so have some of the side-effects become more serious. Therefore, the most able physicians are those who use treatments that have been shown to do more good than harm. Fortunately, modern physicians—and increasingly aware consumers—are asking for proof that a treatment is necessary, and that the outcome is likely to be better than it would have been with no treatment.

Rehabilitation is the fourth critical area of skill. Some problems, like asthma or cerebral palsy, are "chronic" and can't be cured—we just have to live with them. An able doctor tries to rehabilitate a child with a chronic problem, to enable the child to live with as few limitations as possible. In the case of asthma, medication given when the child is well will usually prevent attacks and allow the child to attend school and play sports. In the case of cerebral palsy, the doctor should know which medical and non-medical consultants can help the child lead as full a life as he or she can.

 How much "availability" should I expect from a doctor?

Children get sick, and parents have anxieties, at all times of the day and night. Most often the experienced parent knows when a problem is a real emergency and the child needs to be seen by a doctor without delay. But parents need time to acquire experience, and they need sources of information. We hope this book will help you determine when it's necessary to call your doctor at 2:00 A.M., or rush to an emergency room; we also hope to give you some advice on what steps you yourself can take to make your child feel better while you're deciding whether to call the doctor.

Nevertheless, most parents, no matter how experienced and knowledgeable they are, will need to get in touch with their doctor sometime because their child has an acute problem. And that's when accessibility becomes crucial. Even during office hours, a very busy doctor may be hard to reach because the telephone is constantly in use. Many physicians get around this by having extra telephone lines, so parents can always get through.

Of course, the big problem with availability comes during nights, weekends, and holidays. We recently did a study of after-hours availability in four major Canadian cities. We made phone calls after office hours to doctors who look after children—family physicians and pediatricians—and took note of the messages left on their answering machines or voice mail. We classified a physician as available when the message said that the caller should leave a name and telephone number and that either this physician or the on-call (substitute) physician would reply shortly. When the message said that the office was closed and the patient should be taken to the nearest emergency room or walk-in clinic, we counted the physician as not available after hours.

We found quite a difference in the four cities. In one city, almost all the doctors were available; in another, about three-quarters were not available.

Physician availability gives parents a sense of security, and it's also important for other reasons. A telephone discussion between the parent and a physician solves the majority of after-hours problems; the physician gets enough information to decide whether the child needs to be seen at once, and in more than half the calls, the decision is that there is no need for a doctor to see the child. This not only saves money for the health-care system, but also spares the family a lot of trouble and lost time. Furthermore, each episode successfully handled with after-hours telephone consultation helps give parents the experience and knowledge they need to become less dependent on the health-care system.

No parent can expect a physician to be on call twenty-four hours a day, seven days a week. Years ago many physicians did practice this way, making housecalls, creating a special bond of caring between themselves and the families they served. Although they didn't have many effective treatments to offer, they demonstrated a helping mission that was in itself often therapeutic. Nowadays doctors have many effective treatments to offer, but until fairly recently medical schools concentrated on the curing, not the caring, aspects of being a doctor. That is now changing, as medical educators try to develop an appropriate balance of curing and caring in selecting and educating future doctors.

Most "available" doctors these days practise in on-call groups; this approach enables patients to obtain immediate advice, and doctors to have time for their personal lives. A physician who does not provide an after-hours on-call service, whose message is "Go to the emergency department," should not be your first choice.

Why does "affability" matter in a doctor?

Webster's defines "affable" as "easy to speak to; approachable." We use "affability" to mean the quality that makes you feel at ease talking with a physician—confident that you aren't being rushed out, that the doctor really is interested in discussing your concerns. This climate of interest should be apparent in all office staff—the receptionist, nurse, and others in the practice.

There are several ways the doctor and staff can demonstrate their interest and concern. One is the office setting itself. Although it need not be luxurious, it should at least be pleasant and comfortable, particularly the waiting area. There should be interesting, up-to-date reading material for readers of all ages, as well as toys and games for younger children. The most important components of affability, however, are the interpersonal skills of the doctor and staff, and the feeling that you are not being processed on an assembly line.

The interpersonal skills should include friendliness and the demonstration of a genuine affection for children. Also, the physician should use language the child understands. Often a child can help in arriving at a diagnosis. For example, if a nine-year-old has recurrent tummy aches, the doctor may ask the parent if there is any constipation—a common cause of abdominal pain. But the parent may have no idea of the child's bowel habits, and the child may not understand what "constipation" means. If the doctor asks the child, "Does your tush hurt when you poo?" and the answer is yes, the problem may be solved.

This easy communication should exist at all stages of the system. When you telephone for information or an appointment, you should be made to feel that your request is as important to the doctor and staff as it is to you. When you are seeing the doctor with your child, you should be made to feel that you can discuss anything you wish and that the doctor won't consider it frivolous. When a test is being ordered, you should feel free to ask why it's being done and how the results of the test will affect your child's treatment. You should never leave the office with questions you would have liked to ask. In fact, the affable doctor will usually ask if you have any unanswered questions, or anything else you would like to discuss, before you leave.

The best physicians combine ability with availability and affability. Although these are also the doctors with fairly large practices, they usually have excellent time-management skills, and the people in their care don't feel rushed.

Finding an able, available, and affable doctor for your child

1. Talk to friends, relatives, and neighbors about the physicians who have looked after their children. Ask about the quality of care given, not only by the physician, but by the nurse and receptionist. Is it easy to get through to the office, or is the line always busy? Are the people friendly? Is the office child-oriented? Does the night and weekend message refer to a walk-in clinic or emergency room, or does it pass your number to an on-call physician? Get the names and numbers of the three or four physicians who sound best to you.
2. Call the offices of these physicians on nights and weekends. If the message is to leave your name and number so that a doctor can call you back, keep that physician's name on the list. If not, scratch it off.
3. Visit the office of the physician who ranks highest on your list. In making the appointment, tell the truth: you are looking for a physician for your child, and you would like to meet the doctor, even though your child is currently healthy, or is not yet born. During your visit, assess the office, the staff, and the general atmosphere. If your own opinion agrees with the "word of mouth," you've probably found the right doctor.

Should I look for a pediatrician, or a family doctor?

In some communities there's no choice—the only health-care practitioners available for children are family physicians, who are trained to look after the entire family. The amount of training they have in pediatrics (care of children) varies. Generally, they will have had an average of two months of pediatrics, but many see a lot of children during their two-year training program. Pediatricians are specialists who have had at least four years of training specifically involving children.

Many pediatricians who go into practice become specialists or consultants—that is, they will see only children referred to them by a family physician.

Another level of medical professional is the nurse practitioner—a nurse who has extra training in diagnosis and treatment. Although nurse practitioners are well established in the United States, the profession is in its infancy in

Canada. Most Canadian nurse practitioners work together with physicians, not independently.

But if I can choose either a family physician or a pediatrician as my child's primary health-care provider, which is better?

There's no easy answer, but there have been some studies comparing the ability and availability of the two. In one study, family doctors ordered more unnecessary blood tests than did pediatricians. In another, family doctors gave more unnecessary antibiotics than did pediatricians. A third study showed that children with asthma were less likely to be readmitted to the hospital with an asthma attack if they were examined by a pediatrician than if by a family doctor. In several large Canadian cities, pediatricians were more likely to provide after-hours availability than were family doctors—but the reverse was true in another city.

Of course, these studies apply only to large groups; they don't tell you anything about an individual pediatrician or family doctor. Some family doctors order *fewer* unnecessary tests and treatments, and some are *more* available after hours. It's up to you to get recommendations from people you trust, and to assess those important "three A's"—ability, availability, and affability—to find the right doctor for your child. Good luck!

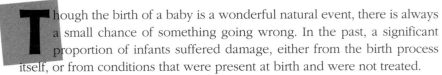

CHAPTER 2

Your Child at Birth

• •

T hough the birth of a baby is a wonderful natural event, there is always a small chance of something going wrong. In the past, a significant proportion of infants suffered damage, either from the birth process itself, or from conditions that were present at birth and were not treated.

These days we have a wide selection of tests, treatments, and procedures that can be used before, during, and after delivery to give a newborn the best possible start. But some parents feel that in focusing on medical aspects of birth, hospitals have intruded too far into what is usually an uncomplicated, joyous family event. The trend now is towards maintaining the intimate family connections of birth as far as possible, while still taking precautions and being prepared for the unforeseen.

Where should babies be born: at home, in a hospital, or in a birthing center?

It's well documented that 85 to 90 percent of deliveries are full-term and uneventful. The remaining 10 to 15 percent involve some sort of complication, but most can be predicted prior to labor, or in the first stage of labor, and appropriate preparations can be made—such as having an obstetrician, a pediatrician/neonatologist (specialist in newborns), and a respiratory therapist present at the delivery. The worrisome cases are those in which the complication doesn't occur until the second stage of labor, when the cervix is fully dilated and delivery is imminent. These late complications include compression or prolapse (early expulsion) of the umbilical cord, premature separation of the placenta, obstructed delivery, and bleeding. Any one of these can reduce the amount of oxygen reaching the baby's brain, which could have serious permanent effects. When one of these complications arises in a hospital, skilled, well-equipped caregivers are on hand to provide immediate help. But if something like this happens in the home, or even in a "stand alone" birthing center, there can be significant delay in treating the baby.

However, most hospitals are sympathetic to parents who want to share their child's birth in a warm, homelike setting rather than in a sterile delivery room. Their compromise has been to install cosy, cheerful "birthing rooms" close to the standard labor and operating rooms, where equipment and personnel are available in case of emergency. If delivery is to be outside a hospital, by a family doctor or midwife, be sure provisions have been made for immediate help if any unforeseen circumstances arise.

 What steps are taken once the baby is born?

The nose and mouth of the baby are cleared of body fluids, the umbilical cord is clamped and cut, and the baby is moved to a special resuscitation table under a heat lamp and is dried off, to prevent heat loss; there can be serious problems in infants who have been stressed by cold at birth. The nose and throat are suctioned to further clear the airway. When the infant is about one minute old, an assessment called an Apgar test is carried out. If the score is below 7, various resuscitative measures are undertaken. These may range from supplying oxygen through a mask to passing a breathing tube down the baby's airway, massaging the heart, using medication to stimulate the heart, and supplying intravenous fluids and drugs. At five min-

Scoring the Apgar test

Sign	Points		
	0	1	2
Color	pale/blue	pink with blue extremities	pink body
Heart rate	not detected	below 100	over 100
Irritability	no response	grimace	lusty cry
Muscle tone	flaccid	some movement	vigorous
Breathing	none	slow, irregular	normal

utes of age, another Apgar assessment is carried out, to tell the doctor or midwife if further resuscitative measures and closer observation are needed.

At this point a brief physical examination is carried out by the doctor or midwife, and nurse in attendance. An identification band is placed around the baby's ankle or wrist, drops or ointment (usually erythromycin or silver nitrate) are put in the eyes to prevent infection by organisms called "gonococcus" and "chlamydia," and an injection of vitamin K is given in the thigh to prevent a serious condition called "hemorrhagic (bleeding) disease of the newborn." Then, if the baby has adapted well to life outside the womb, he or she is handed to the parents to hold—often for skin-to-skin contact and preliminary suckling at the mother's breast.

What should a newborn look like?

When you have your first chance to see your new baby, you may notice a few variations from normal. Most newborns are, quite frankly, a bit ugly (except to Mom and Dad!). A baby born a few weeks early is often covered with fine hair called "lanugo" (this will disappear in a week or two) and may have a thick cheesy material, the *vernix caseosa*, over much of the body (this will be removed during the first bath). If the baby has had a bit of oxygen shortage during labor, there is occasionally some sticky dark green or black material from the bowels, called "meconium," on the skin. You may notice some pearly white or yellow spots on the face, called "milia" (sebaceous gland hyperplasia), which look like pimples or pustules—these will disappear in a few weeks. Some infants develop a fluctuating whole-body rash called "erythema toxicum," which resembles little pimples with red rims— this too will be gone in a few days without treatment. Many normal newborns have some degree of cyanosis (blue color) in their hands and feet and around the mouth, due to their immature blood circulation. You may notice that your baby's head has a weird shape, especially if you had a long, difficult labor; this is caused by molding during the birth process, especially at the back ("cone head"), and is called "caput succedaneum." You may see a fluctuating mass at one side of the head, not crossing the mid-line, caused by some bleeding under the scalp, called a "cephalhematoma." The odd shape will disappear in days, and the scalp bulge in a few weeks. You may notice that your baby looks bow-legged and that his or her feet turn in; this is due to the baby's position in the womb, and will gradually correct itself by about age two.

Will the baby be kept in a nursery?

Most hospitals now allow healthy newborn infants to "room in" with their mothers, as long as there are no concerns or complications that require monitoring in the neonatal intensive care unit. The assigned nurse is trained to look after both the mother and her baby, and to teach the parents the basics of infant care—especially to help get breast-feeding established. The physician or midwife will carry out a more complete examination of the baby within twenty-four hours, answer any questions, and arrange follow-up after discharge. There will be another examination if the hospital stay is more than forty-eight hours.

How much can a newborn do?

Your new baby's nervous system has a number of unique features, many of which help an infant adapt to the outside world. These are called "primitive reflexes." One is the Moro or "startle" reflex: a sudden noise or disturbance will cause the baby's arms and hands to open and move in a sort of embrace. The suckling reflex is another, as is the rooting reflex: if the infant's cheek is brushed, the baby turns to face that side and suckles (this is important to know when you're breast-feeding). There's the grasp reflex: when an object is placed in the baby's hand, the hand automatically closes over it; and the walking reflex: when the infant is held upright with the feet just touching a surface, one foot after the other will be placed down, simulating walking. As well, the infant is able to fix his or her eyes on special, interesting, close-up objects such as a parent's face. Except for this last one, these primitive reflexes gradually disappear by nine months of age.

What other tests are done in hospital?

Throughout most of the United States and Canada newborns are screened for two diseases that, if not detected and treated in the first two or three weeks of life, can result in severe and permanent mental retardation. These diseases are congenital hypothyroidism—"CH" (1 case per 4,500 births)—and phenylketonuria—"PKU" (1 case per 12,000 births). Some jurisdictions screen for a number of other diseases as well: galactosemia, homocystinuria, sickle cell anemia, congenital adrenal hyperplasia, biotinidase deficiency, maple syrup urine disease, cystic fibrosis, muscular dystrophy, etc. Whereas everyone agrees on the value of CH and PKU screening, the value and cost-effectiveness of these other tests has not yet been established.

The CH and PKU tests may not be reliable if carried out in the first few hours of life, so experts generally recommend that the infant be over twenty-four hours old when they are performed. If the baby goes home before that, the test can be done at discharge and repeated two or three days later. (These policies may change as new information emerges.) It's most important that all babies have these two screening tests, at the appropriate age, since early diagnosis is critical and cannot be made by a simple physical exam.

Why do some newborns look yellowish?

Jaundice—yellowing of a baby's skin and eyeballs—is very common; 60 to 70 percent of full-term newborns show some visible jaundice. In the great majority of cases it's a harmless normal variation (physiological jaundice) and needs no special treatment. Physiological jaundice appears after twenty-four hours of age and is more common in premature, Asian, and breast-fed infants. The yellow color comes from a pigment called "bilirubin," and is thought to be due to delayed maturing of the chemical processes in the liver that break down the normal end-products of red blood cells. There is controversy as to whether this type of jaundice is ever dangerous; very occasional adverse results have been reported. The most common treatment is a procedure called "phototherapy," in which the infant is placed in an incubator or special blanket and exposed to certain wavelengths of light that decrease the jaundice. This sometimes results in a couple of extra days in hospital or, rarely, readmission.

Sometimes, however, the accumulation of bilirubin is caused by specific disease processes (pathological jaundice) and can lead to serious consequences. The one doctors worry about most is called "kernicterus" and involves damage to the brain resulting in hearing loss, mental retardation, and certain types of cerebral palsy, or even death. Kernicterus is now fortunately quite rare. Pathological jaundice often appears in less than twenty-four hours and can be the result of a large number of causes, including mother–infant blood incompatibility; bacterial infection; and various metabolic, viral, or structural diseases of the liver. The physician must be aware of all the possibilities and begin appropriate tests in a timely fashion. Treatment may include an exchange transfusion, in which most of the infant's blood is temporarily replaced and the bilirubin is removed. Great care is now given to ensure that blood and blood products are free of infectious agents such as HIV and the hepatitis virus. Even so, doctors are very careful to do exchange transfusions only when the baby's life or brain is at risk.

The debate over circumcision

Routine male newborn circumcision (surgical removal of the foreskin) is a very controversial, often emotional subject. Some families and physicians are vehemently opposed, while others are strongly in favor. In 1989 the American Academy of Pediatrics task force on neonatal circumcision adopted a revised policy that the procedure "has potential medical benefits and advantages as well as disadvantages and risks." For details on these, see Chapter 8, "Painful Urination." The Canadian Paediatric Society's official statement is that it is an "unnecessary procedure," though the society admits that 5 percent of those not circumcised at birth will need to have the procedure done later because of medical complications.

Some health plans have delisted routine newborn circumcision; in such cases both the physician and the hospital will charge you to perform the procedure. You should therefore check the cost as well as discussing the pros and cons with your doctor.

 How long should a newborn and mother stay in hospital?

Governments are wrestling with the spiraling cost of health care and the diminishing dollars available to pay for it. One of the strategies for reducing hospital costs is early discharge of the normal newborn; most normal full-term babies and their mothers are now discharged after forty-eight hours, and there is a very strong push to reduce this to twenty-four hours, although there is talk of legislation to reverse this trend. Early discharge is of concern to neonatologists and pediatricians since it may interfere with the appropriate timing for CH and PKU blood tests, and since some of the more common problems don't become obvious until the second or third day of life—for example, jaundice, congenital heart disease, infection, certain genetic metabolic diseases, and feeding problems. In addition, it's difficult to teach a mother and her family how to care for and breast-feed a baby in such a short time. This is the reason for the new recommendation that the first well-baby visit by the physician or midwife should take place three or four days after discharge.

Many obstetrical/neonatal units have introduced programs incorporating prenatal and postnatal classes not only about pregnancy and delivery, but also about breast-feeding; formula feeding; bathing; cord care; and how to manage crying, sleeping, fever, bowel problems, spitting up, skin care, etc. Most of these programs cost extra, but you should consider them, even if you are an experienced parent with lots of family support. All of these topics are covered in detail in this book.

What happens when a baby is born prematurely?

Preterm birth is usually defined as less than thirty-seven weeks' gestation, with birth weight less than 5.5 pounds (2.5 kg). Premature babies previously had significant risks of chest diseases and brain damage; in the last twenty years, however, these risks have lessened substantially. Now, with proper care, many premature babies with a gestational age as low as twenty-eight weeks and a birth weight as low as 2.2 pounds (1 kg) grow into normal children.

If the premature baby is doing well as far as breathing and feeding are concerned, and if the birth weight is not too low (at least 4 pounds or 1.8 kg,), the baby is usually not transferred to a special care nursery or neonatal intensive care unit. Once there is a reasonable weight gain (⅓ to 1 ounce, 10 to 30 gm, per day for at least three days), and the baby has no difficulty maintaining normal pink color and normal body temperature on his or her own, the baby may be discharged. If there are breathing and/or feeding problems, or if the weight is less than 4 lb, referral to a special care nursery, where there are specially trained staff and technology such as respirators, may be necessary. The duration of stay in the special care nursery depends on how long it takes the baby to breathe normally and gain weight appropriately; it varies from weeks to months.

What do I do about the cord after I go home?

The umbilical cord should be gently cleaned at the base several times daily with a cotton-tipped applicator soaked in alcohol. It will fall off in four to six days if it dries quickly, and in seven to ten days if it remains a bit moist. If the skin around the cord becomes inflamed or if there is an odor or a discharge of pus, call your physician.

The baby's first bath should always be carried out under the supervision of an experienced person. Daily bathing can be at any convenient time, except immediately after the baby's feeding. Sponge baths are usually recommended until the cord falls off; then the infant can be immersed in the tub.

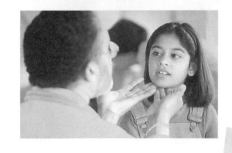

CHAPTER 3

You and the Doctor: Working Together

• •

Once your baby is born, one of the important rituals of parenting is the well-child visit. Each appointment serves as a milestone marking your child's progress. Probably before you realize it, your little baby will have become a teenager who presents you with a new set of concerns just as challenging as those of infancy. Regularly scheduled checkups provide an excellent opportunity to review your child's growth, current development, and future needs, both physical and emotional. These visits also offer you a chance to deal with any doubts or concerns you may have.

What happens at a well-child visit?

Each checkup is unique, as its contents depend upon your child's age. Yet the goals of all these health-maintenance visits are much the same. The doctor wants to identify and help treat any physical, developmental, or behavioral problems that may exist, so a careful medical history and physical examination are part of every checkup. Certain screening tests, such as for tuberculosis, may be performed. The doctor may provide counseling on more general topics, such as nutrition and accident prevention. Any specific concerns that remain unanswered are addressed. Finally, immunizations are discussed and administered according to the recommended guidelines.

How often should I take my child for a well-child visit?

During infancy, your baby will experience a number of remarkable changes over just a few months. Because you need to keep abreast of these developments, and to ensure proper immunization, you will visit your baby's doctor regularly during this period. Ideally the frequency of these visits will result in a successful relationship; the better your communication is with the doctor, the better your child's care is likely to be. As your child grows older, the intervals between well-child visits grow longer.

When do I start these visits?

Until recently, a new mother would spend a number of days in hospital recovering from childbirth and learning how to care for her newborn; now most mothers and babies go home after just a day or two. The comfort of being in your own home is undoubtedly welcome, but a number of issues must be addressed. For example, it's unlikely that breast-feeding will be established in the first forty-eight hours. Most parents are concerned that their infant isn't getting enough milk; others fear that the baby is too jaundiced. On a few occasions, these worries are justified. Obviously, it's better to nip any problems in the bud. Thus it is recommended that the first office visit be scheduled for the baby's first week of life, especially if the baby has been discharged from the hospital early.

At this first visit, you will be encouraged to tell your doctor how you're feeling, not only about your baby, but also about the demands of parenting. Suggestions to help with breast-feeding will be offered, if needed. The doctor will ask about the frequency of the baby's urination and, if you have a little boy, the force of the urinary stream, since a poor stream may be an early sign of obstruction. Stooling patterns will also be reviewed. Your baby will be weighed, measured, and carefully examined for any late-presenting birth defect. Your physician will advise you of normal patterns of sleep and feeding; most newborns sleep for about three hours at a stretch and are then wakeful for about an hour, wanting to be fed. You should discuss child-safety issues related to sleep position, crib safety, and bathwater temperature. If your child is to receive the hepatitis vaccine in infancy, the first dose will be given at this time, if it wasn't administered in hospital.

At the end of this first checkup, some well-deserved words of encouragement will generally be offered. You may also be reminded to try to pace yourself a bit. *Parenting is not a sprint—it's a marathon!*

How long should I wait before the next visit?

Your doctor will probably suggest that visits take place every few months; a typical pattern would be a visit at two, four, six, nine, twelve, fifteen, and eighteen months.

The two-month visit: By now, your baby will display the distinctive behavior and temperament that make him or her a unique individual. Although you

Sudden infant death syndrome (SIDS)

SIDS, or "crib death," is a tragic disorder that causes the sudden, totally unexpected death of an apparently healthy infant, usually between one and four months of age. It seems that the children just stop breathing, often while asleep; first aid will not revive them. Studies have suggested some contributing factors to SIDS, but we still don't understand exactly what goes wrong. It does not seem to be genetic.

But while the unpredictability and mystery of SIDS are frightening to parents of young infants, the condition is rare in North America. In fact, as more is learned about the disorder, it appears some of the deaths attributed to SIDS in the past were in fact due to other causes.

Our understanding of SIDS is developing rapidly. Ask your doctor for the latest information on risks for this disorder, and keep in mind that secondhand smoke appears to be a factor. But try not to dwell on the threat; despite all the press coverage, the risk of crib death is very low.

may not yet feel like an expert on child care, you certainly know more about your own baby than anybody else does.

This is an important time to discuss your comfort level with parenting. If your child is having irregular feeding or sleeping patterns, if the baby is colicky, or if you feel tired and overwhelmed, share those feelings. That way, you and your doctor can manage them as a team.

Once again, your baby will be weighed and measured to make certain that growth is satisfactory, and examined for appropriate responsiveness. Any new problems, such as thrush or diaper rash, will be addressed (see Chapter 10, "Skin: Spots and Rashes"). You will likely be advised that night waking is still to be expected, and that you shouldn't rush the introduction of solid foods. Finally, after a discussion of the advantages and potential side-effects, the baby will receive immunizations against diphtheria, tetanus, and pertussis (a DTP shot), polio, and *Haemophilus influenzae* type B (Hib). The second hepatitis B vaccine will also be administered.

The four-month visit: By now, your baby should appear curious about the world, and eager to be part of it. The doctor will check that developmental changes are progressing on schedule. As in all well-baby visits, a careful physical examination will be done to identify any health problems.

Most children are ready for the introduction of solids between four and

Typical immunization patterns

Disease	1st shot or series	1st booster	2nd booster	Further boosters
Diphtheria, tetanus, pertussis (DTP)	2, 4, & 6 months	18 months	school entry	
Tetanus & diphtheria (Td)				age 14 & every 10 years
Haemophilus influenzae type B (Hib)	2, 4, & 6 months (with DTP)	15–18 months		
Measles, mumps, & rubella (MMR)	12–15 months	4–6 years, or in pre-adolescence		
Polio (shots)	2, 4, & 6 months (with DTP)	18 months	age 4	every 10 years
Polio (oral)	2 & 4 months	18 months	school entry	
Chicken pox	A vaccine has been approved in the United States but, as of 1996, is not approved in Canada. The first dose is usually given with MMR. If the first dose is given in the teen years, a booster is needed 4 to 8 weeks later.			
Hepatitis B	Vaccination is recommended but the ideal age remains uncertain. One schedule advises a shot just after birth, with a booster at 1 month and another between 6 and 18 months. Another suggests 3 doses, starting in preadolescence.			

six months of age, so you will be discussing how best to accomplish this. (See Chapter 12, "Feeding Your Child.")

Because most infants are starting to reach and roll by this age, safety at the change table will be highlighted. Next, it's time for immunizations again. You will review how the last shots were tolerated, and then the second DTP, Hib, and polio vaccines will be given. Before you leave, be sure to ask any questions you may still have.

Secondhand smoke and your child

Parents who smoke have usually tried stopping—even before becoming parents. There are certain risks to children exposed to secondhand smoke that parents should be aware of. The possibility of sudden infant death syndrome (SIDS, also called crib death) is greater in young infants exposed to secondhand smoke. The risk of recurrent ear infections is also greater. Finally, children with asthma may have more attacks when exposed to secondhand smoke. Sometimes just knowing what their smoking may do to their children is enough for parents to get the help they need from their doctor to quit. If you can't quit, try not to smoke in your home or close to your child.

The six-month visit: By now, you're probably feeling quite comfortable with parenting. Although time seems to have flown by, chances are you barely remember when you weren't a parent. You may be thinking of returning to work outside the home, or you may have already done so. Thus this visit may be a good time to discuss what to look for in day care or a babysitter. Other issues usually addressed at this visit include teething and sleep problems. Teething seems the most variable and, arguably, the least important of infant milestones; most children get their first tooth around this time, but others appear in no rush. A few children are still waking in the night, while others who used to sleep through have reverted to getting up. The six-month checkup is a good time to review normal childhood sleep patterns and develop effective strategies for any sleep disturbance. (See Chapter 9, "Sleeping Patterns and Problems.") After the physical examination, the third DTP/Hib immunization will be given. If your baby is receiving inactivated polio vaccine, the third dose will be administered with the same injection. The final hepatitis B shot will be given to those infants who received the earlier two doses. During this visit, you may discuss safety issues such as infant walkers and the danger of small objects reaching a baby's mouth.

The nine-month visit: This visit coincides with rapid developmental change. Instead of needing the world to be brought within reach, the infant acquires the mobility to explore everything, with great curiosity. The thrust of this visit will be to evaluate how well your baby is acquiring these motor skills, and how sociable and communicative he or she has become.

Although child-safety advice is a feature of most well-baby visits, the nine-month checkup in particular tries to guarantee that mobility will lead to discovery and not tragedy. The use of stairway gates and the dangers of electrical cords will likely be discussed. Since the nine-month examination covers the introduction of finger foods, the risk of choking on certain foods may be pointed out. The visit should prompt a thorough review of household safety.

No vaccinations are required at this visit. Many doctors perform a tuberculin test, especially if there are factors that increase the probability of infection. Other physicians check the hemoglobin level for iron-deficiency anemia, but this condition is declining in frequency in infancy, and there is now doubt as to whether every child requires a routine hemoglobin test.

The twelve-month visit: Where did the time go? Your baby is rapidly becoming a walking, talking, and increasingly independent individual. He or she seems capable of more sustained and focused play, and has learned to assert himself or herself in an organized fashion. Simple words begin to have meaning. It's an exciting time for both children and their parents.

The twelve-month visit attempts to verify that these developments are progressing satisfactorily. Your doctor will also ask about the successful transition from purées to table foods. The introduction of cow's milk and the transition to a cup will likely be discussed. Dental care, especially the need to avoid bottles of milk in the crib, will be highlighted.

The injection to prevent measles, mumps, and rubella—the MMR vaccine—will be given either at this visit or at fifteen months.

The fifteen-month visit: Once again, your baby will be measured, weighed, and examined to check that physical growth is progressing satisfactorily. By now, protection from maternal antibodies has worn off and the baby has been exposed to a variety of germs in places such as day care. How he or she has dealt with these early-childhood illnesses will be reviewed.

Development will again be assessed. Most children are walking, using their fingers to feed themselves, handling a cup, and starting to use a few words by this time. Some are showing their assertiveness very clearly: their ability to protest loudly may have become a finely developed skill!

Immunizations will be reviewed, and those children who have yet to receive their MMR shot will be vaccinated.

The eighteen-month visit: At this checkup, the emphasis will be on dealing with your toddler's emerging autonomy. It's important to realize that strong food preferences will likely have developed. Try to remember that a dislike of broccoli is not fatal. If your child seems to hate vegetables, he or she is not alone. Your physician will likely point out that a child of this age doesn't require huge quantities of food. It's best to present a balanced diet, and to avoid too much milk or juice.

Autonomy will also be an issue when it comes to discipline. Children at this age resist limits, however reasonable they may seem. Yet establishing consistent, reasonable limits is important for your happiness as well as your child's. Developing bedtime routines and strategies for dealing with temper tantrums will be well worth the effort.

At this age, a number of children are beginning to show an interest in toiletting. It's best not to rush things, but if your youngster seems aware of these bodily functions, it's reasonable to review toilet training with your doctor to avoid some of the pitfalls that occasionally lead to frustration.

Immunizations are again required. The booster for diphtheria, tetanus, pertussis, polio, and Hib are all administered.

 ### How long do I continue these frequent well-baby visits?

Your next health-maintenance visit will likely be at two years, and after that a single annual examination should be sufficient to monitor your youngster's needs. Nonetheless, you and your doctor may remain in close contact; a number of toddlers develop one ear infection or bout of wheezing after another. Since a needle is no longer an inevitable part of each visit, your child may actually start looking forward to coming to the doctor.

The two-year visit: Developmental issues will likely dominate this checkup. By this stage the toddler is acquiring increasing verbal skills. Most have learned fifty words or more and are using short phrases such as "What's that?" Your physician will ask how your child is progressing in this regard, and answer any questions about diet. The use of a toothbrush, at least in imitation of other family members, may be encouraged. You will likely discuss toilet training at this time.

Perhaps the greatest parental challenge at this stage lies in discipline; it's quite a chore teaching a youngster to harness impulses. You may want to review how best to establish limits and handle temper tantrums. This age does not have to be the "Terrible Twos."

Often, at this visit, parents seek their doctor's opinion about preschool programs. Keep in mind that the important part of a toddler's curriculum is not gymnastics, painting, or swimming, but developing the social skills to get along well with others.

The three-year visit: At this visit the doctor will assess how well your child is acquiring the developmental skills needed to function well in the world outside your home. By now, children should be talking in short sentences. For many youngsters at this stage, ideas come more rapidly than they can be expressed: stuttering is common but, fortunately, is usually temporary. Toilet training has been achieved in about 90 percent of three-year-olds, which is a blessing. Furthermore, discipline is usually managed with less of a struggle than previously, as the concept of consequences begins to sink in. If any of these areas of development presents concerns, they should be addressed at this visit.

Sleep problems may still be an issue, but generally the cause is different. The earlier sleep disorders reflect separation anxiety, whereas now the problem may be a very vivid imagination. A three-year-old's fantasy world seems as real as the actual one. A little one may need some help dealing with the monsters and demons that tend to crop up in nightmares.

As before, height and weight will be recorded, and a physical examination carried out. Girls of this age often complain of vaginal discomfort, perhaps because of inefficient early attempts at toileting. This problem should be sensitively managed. In addition, an attempt will be made to assess both vision and blood pressure more accurately. By the end of this examination, your child may actually enjoy having a checkup.

The preschool examination: This visit occurs around the time of kindergarten entry, when the child is four or five years old. Although it's a complete exam, the prime focus is on school readiness. How well a child sees (including color differentiation), how well he or she listens, and how the fine motor skills have developed will all be carefully assessed. Guidelines on watching television may also be discussed.

This checkup will also focus on the child's general maturity, activity level, and temperament. You will describe how your youngster plays with other children, responds to discipline and limits, and accepts separation from parents, and whether his or her general approach to situations is a positive or negative one.

The child-safety issues mentioned will reflect this stage of increased independence. Does your child know your address and telephone number? Is he or she prepared to respond to strangers appropriately?

At this visit, a booster for diphtheria, tetanus, pertussis, and polio will be given. A tuberculin skin test may be administered as well, if there is a chance your child has had contact with a person with tuberculosis.

 ### Once my child is in school, do these exams continue?

Many doctors continue health-maintenance visits on an annual basis. It's crucial that a child's early educational experience be as successful as possible, and most parents view their physician as part of the team working to achieve that goal. Increasingly, pediatric training places great emphasis on both childhood learning and the management of educational difficulties. Your physician will see himself or herself as an advocate for your youngster, so don't hesitate to share any concerns about education, behavior, or attention span.

A physical examination will still be performed. At this stage, most children—male or female—tend to be quite shy about being examined. This is natural, and your doctor will respond sensitively.

Athletics tend to become more and more important at this age. You may discuss community sports programs and enrolling your child in swim classes; you will likely talk about bicycle safety and in-line skating. Far too many children die needlessly, or suffer serious injury, because basic safety precautions have been overlooked or rejected.

These checkups continue into the preadolescent years. Many pediatricians and family doctors look forward to visits more at this stage than at any other. Their young patients seem healthier and are in the office less frequently, so the well-child visits help firm the bonds between the doctor and the child. Children at this age are usually terrific—enthusiastic about their team sports and all extracurricular activities. Energy and creativity abound, and their *joie de vivre* is infectious.

Sometimes, however, this stage is not the bed of roses it should be. Difficulties at school, troubles with peers, and coping with parental separation or remarriage can cloud a child's emotions. If a youngster appears to be struggling with a problem, this visit may serve as a catalyst to seeking a solution.

The physical examination includes the continued monitoring of height and weight. Vision is checked again, as nearsightedness may appear at this age. Any early signs of puberty will be noted and reassurance provided, particularly to young boys who notice firm little lumps under their nipples (this is simply breast tissue, which will disappear over time). The spine will be checked for abnormal curvature, which appears first in preadolescence.

Immunization practices vary at this stage, depending upon local policies.

Some children receive the series of inoculations to protect against hepatitis B. Many physicians provide a booster dose for measles, mumps, and rubella as part of the visit.

What about the teen years?

Adolescence presents a challenge for both parents and physicians. Sometimes it helps to remember that this period is turbulent for the adolescent as well. It's a time of great change, both physically and behaviorally. When we are children, for better or worse, our value system depends largely upon that of our parents. Adults, on the other hand, should have a clear idea of who they are and what is really important to them. The transformation from child to adult, during which unwanted values are discarded and replaced by the young person's own adult choices, constitutes the great developmental task of adolescence. The whole process necessarily involves experimentation and rebellion. Most teens, if they are honest with themselves, find the period difficult and unsettling.

Health-maintenance visits during adolescence should be framed by these realities. A frank discussion about confidentiality and privacy is usually a good idea, and both the parents and the adolescent should be involved. Patient care tends to be best when good communication exists between the physician and the patient. This can be more easily accomplished when the teenage patient trusts that any discussion will be confidential. With this privilege comes some degree of responsibility: it should be the adolescent's job to attend appointments on time. Like most dealings with teenagers, the visits will be less stressful if the rules and policies are discussed in advance and found to be mutually agreeable.

Much of the physical examination of teens during their health-maintenance visits tends to deal with issues of puberty. For females, this involves monitoring the onset of menstruation and possibly managing irregular or painful periods. A clear and open-ended invitation to discuss contraception should be issued to the teenager. Most physicians try to handle the issues related to adolescent sexuality in a non-threatening and supportive fashion.

In early adolescence, a number of children, especially boys, lag behind their peers in both growth and sexual maturation. This can be quite troubling; it's hard on a child to look ten years old when some classmates can pass for seventeen. It's also a challenge to compete athletically with such a size disadvantage. Fortunately, time is a great equalizer, and catch-up growth is the rule.

The teen is still weighed and measured on each checkup. Some diseases—inflammatory bowel disease, for example—begin very gradually, and poor weight gain can be the first sign. The weight check will also provide an opportunity to discuss another problem of adolescence: eating disorders. How teens perceive their size and shape, and what they eat, are important topics that should be addressed during these visits.

A number of other physical issues are particularly important to the adolescent. What teens see in the mirror is not what the rest of us notice. Acne is perceived as a curse more dreadful than the great plagues, and working out an effective but not excessive treatment plan is one of the goals at teen examinations. These visits also serve the adolescent athlete, who is usually required to undergo a physical exam before participating in a team sport.

What about the adolescent with a chronic illness or disability? Most teens with an ongoing problem simply wish their disease would disappear so they could be like everyone else. One response they sometimes fall into is ignoring some or even all of their treatment. It's crucial for the doctor to let the teenager vent his or her feelings about living with asthma, diabetes, epilepsy, or whatever the chronic problem happens to be. If possible, the patient with a chronic illness must be persuaded that complying with the treatment plan is the best way to ensure as normal a life as possible.

 ## Do teenagers get immunizations too?

Upon entry into high school, teens receive a booster for tetanus and diphtheria. If the inactivated polio vaccine was used earlier, another dose will be administered, in combination with the other two vaccines. Furthermore, if the hepatitis B vaccine has not yet been received, the three doses, given over a six-month period, should be administered as early in adolescence as possible.

More teenage girls are taking up smoking than ever before, perhaps because they think that it's "cool" or that it will help them control their weight. Nagging doesn't work, but information about the known risks may. A doctor can explain how smoking reduces cardiovascular fitness. It may also help—especially with girls—to remind them of the strong odor of smoking, and the smelly residue left on hair and clothes.

Many teens don't realize that smoking is more than just a cancer risk; it's also a major risk for heart disease, and lung diseases such as emphysema. The most important factor in cutting down heart disease in the last thirty years has been the fact that many fewer males are smoking than before; it is tragic that this saving of lives is offset by the increase in female smoking.

As with nutrition and exercise, the best argument you can offer is your own example. It's difficult to make a convincing case against smoking with a pack of cigarettes in your pocket!

Again, some advice on safety is in order. Accidental injury, and even death, remain the greatest danger to the well-being of most teenagers. Even if the impact is slight, most physicians feel that providing some advice on safety is a key part of an adolescent's annual exam. (Chapter 13 provides a thorough summary of safety precautions for various ages.) In the later teen years, a candid conversation about alcohol use, particularly in the context of social events, is worthwhile. Even getting a teen to pledge not to ride home with a driver who has been drinking is an important step in promoting responsible behavior. For doctors as well as parents, it's best to remember that with teenagers, discussions work much better than lectures.

 What about side-effects of all these immunizations?

It's hard to imagine a world in which thousands of helpless children suffocated in their own bodily secretions because they had contracted diphtheria, or lay paralysed in an iron-lung machine because of polio, or died of measles-related pneumonia. Yet that is how things were. The development of immunizations has dramatically reduced the occurrence of such preventable tragedies. It remains one of humankind's great achievements.

Still, these miracle preventives can have side-effects—some minor, some serious—as indicated below. For information on the diseases themselves, see Chapter 14, "Diseases and Medical Conditions."

Chicken pox immunization uses a live, attenuated (specially grown and weakened) vaccine that is recommended in the United States for all healthy children after twelve months of age if there is no clear history of prior chicken pox infection. The vaccine is well tolerated, with very few significant side-effects. Five percent of children get a fever ten to fourteen days after inoculation, but only a few of these develop a rash. In teens, a rash is slightly more common.

The **diphtheria** vaccine, diphtheria toxoid, is a preparation of diphtheria toxin inactivated by formaldehyde. Infants generally tolerate the inoculation well, but temporary local reactions and fever may occur. These side-effects are more common in older children, so the vaccine for this age group is adjusted to contain less toxoid.

Hepatitis B immunization uses a vaccine made from genetically engineered purified hepatitis B protein. The vaccine cannot cause hepatitis. No serious complications from the vaccine have been reported in children, but local irritation at the site of the injection, low-grade fever, and irritability occur in approximately 10 percent of cases.

The various **Hib** vaccines appear remarkably safe. Fever and local irritation occur at rates similar to those following injection with a harmless placebo, and no severe life-threatening reactions have been associated with the vaccine.

The vaccines developed to combat **measles, mumps,** and **rubella** are routinely given as a combined MMR injection. They are live, attenuated vaccines, intended to create an infection so mild that no clinical symptoms result and yet lifelong immunity is induced. This protection is obtained in the great majority of children.

Fever and a temporary rash occur in about 10 percent of vaccine recipients, usually around ten days after the inoculation. Sore joints, thought to be due to the rubella component, are occasionally noted after a few weeks, but this is much more likely in older patients, especially women. Other side-effects, ranging from tingling fingers to encephalitis, are extremely rare.

The live MMR vaccines must be given with caution to, or even withheld from, children with immune deficiencies or a sensitivity to certain elements of the vaccines such as neomycin or egg-white. Administration of MMR should be delayed if the child has a severe acute illness, but not for minor acute illness, even if fever is present. There is a growing consensus that a second MMR injection should be given to immunize against measles in particular, to protect the 5 percent of children who fail to respond to the first inoculation and to boost any possible waning immunity in others. Universal, successful immunization may result in total eradication of this disease.

At this time most **pertussis** (whooping cough) vaccine is prepared from a suspension of killed *Bordetella pertussis* organisms. It isn't perfect. First, it's only partially effective; about two-thirds of children receive total protection and 95 percent will be spared the severe forms of the disease if they are exposed to the germ. Furthermore, there is the risk of side-effects, some quite scary. Minor local reactions at the site of the injection, or fever and fussiness, occur in about half the recipients. Fortunately, these problems disappear on their own in a day or two. Rarely, persistent and inconsolable crying that lasts for hours follows pertussis vaccination. Convulsions or a state of limp unresponsiveness have been reported in approximately 1 out of 1,750 recipients. Most of these convulsions are brief and related to fever; neither these nor seizures unaccompanied by fever have been implicated in producing later epilepsy.

There has been widespread fear about a possible association of severe neurological disease and the pertussis vaccine. The problem has been exhaustively studied and debated. Permanent neurological damage does *not* appear to be caused by the vaccine and, if it were, the increased occurrence would be so slight as to be essentially unmeasurable. Note that brain damage, and even death, can result from getting the actual disease.

Any child who has had a severe allergic reaction to the pertussis vaccine should not have another DTP dose. If an episode of reduced responsiveness or marked listlessness occurred shortly after the vaccination, the relative risks of further immunization with DTP must be considered. Although no long-term effects of such an event have been reported, your doctor and you may decide against further inoculation with DTP, particularly if the risk of pertussis is low in your community.

Some conditions that were once felt to be reasons to avoid DTP immunization are no longer considered enough of a risk to interfere with complete vaccination. These include high fever within forty-eight hours of inoculation, persistent crying, or a prior history of seizures that are now controlled. Also, a minor viral illness such as the common cold, even if accompanied by fever, need not delay the vaccination.

If you give your child acetaminophen around the time of injection, side-effects such as fever, irritability, and local reaction will be significantly diminished. In the future, newer types of pertussis vaccine (acellular vaccines) may provide protection with fewer reactions. For now, one thing is clear: children are at greater risk when they remain unimmunized than when they are properly vaccinated.

Two different methods of **polio** protection are available, inactivated (IPV) and live oral (OPV) polio virus vaccine. Both are effective in preventing the disease caused by the three different strains of polio virus. The side-effects of the current IPV shots are minimal and essentially limited to minor local reactions. OPV contains live virus and can cause vaccine-associated paralysis on very rare occasions; the risk to vaccine recipients is estimated at 1 case per 11.7 million doses of distributed vaccine, and the risk to people in contact with those vaccinated is calculated at about 1 case per 3 million doses. OPV should never be administered to immunodeficient children, those on medication that interferes with immunity, or children closely associated with such vulnerable individuals. Immunizing children whose mothers are pregnant, however, presents no risk to the unborn children.

Immunization against **tetanus** is with tetanus toxoid, which is tetanus toxin treated with formaldehyde and combined with an aluminum salt. Adverse reactions to primary immunization are quite rare.

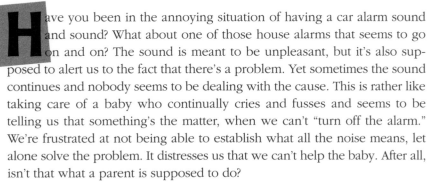

CHAPTER 4

Crying: How Much Is Normal?

Have you been in the annoying situation of having a car alarm sound and sound? What about one of those house alarms that seems to go on and on? The sound is meant to be unpleasant, but it's also supposed to alert us to the fact that there's a problem. Yet sometimes the sound continues and nobody seems to be dealing with the cause. This is rather like taking care of a baby who continually cries and fusses and seems to be telling us that something's the matter, when we can't "turn off the alarm." We're frustrated at not being able to establish what all the noise means, let alone solve the problem. It distresses us that we can't help the baby. After all, isn't that what a parent is supposed to do?

Of course, all babies cry and fuss from time to time. Unfortunately, some of them do so a lot more than others—especially in the first few months of life.

Q How much do most babies cry? At what age do they cry most?

In a study done by the well-known pediatrician Dr. T. Berry Brazelton, eighty mothers were asked to keep daily records of their infants' crying for the first twelve weeks of life. In each twenty-four-hour period, they indicated what the baby was doing at various times (crying, feeding, sleeping, sucking, being held). Whenever the baby cried, they noted the type of cry (sudden or gradual), what relieved it and for how long, and what seemed to have caused it.

Dr. Brazelton chose mothers who seemed to have a normal, positive approach to mothering; more than half had more than one child, were known to him personally, and were described as relaxed and competent.

The study showed that crying increased from an hour and forty-five minutes per day at two weeks of age to a peak of two hours and forty-five minutes at six weeks, and then gradually diminished to less than an hour by twelve weeks.

What time of day do babies cry most?

Dr. Brazelton found that in three-week-old infants, the fussing was spread through the day but there was a strong tendency to cry between 6:00 and 11:00 P.M. By six weeks there was occasional crying in the early morning, but most fussing occurred later in the day; some babies began around noon, many cried between 6:00 and 8:00 P.M., and a few were crying after 2:00 A.M. By ten weeks of age the babies had quieted down considerably; what little crying they did was mostly between 6:00 A.M. and noon, or between 4:30 and 10:30 in the evening.

What's the difference between "fussing" and crying?

When babies cry because they are hungry or wet, you can generally soothe them by solving the problem—with a feeding, a dry diaper, or whatever. The term "fussing" is generally applied to crying that goes on for no apparent reason; the child rejects a pacifier and other proffered solutions, and may quiet briefly if picked up or rocked, but starts crying again when this attention is removed. Fussing is frustrating for parents because they feel that the child must want something, yet they can't figure out what it is.

If that's fussing, then what is "colic"?

"Colic"—sometimes called "three-month colic"—is indicated by a more extreme degree of fussing. It has been described as "bursts of irritability, fussing, or crying lasting for a total of more than three hours a day and occurring on more than three days in any one week, for at least three weeks." But colic also seems to involve a far more intense and angry type of fussing, which is acutely distressing to parents. Mothers can be so upset by the persistent crying of a colicky baby that they begin to lose their milk; the persistent frustration and helplessness can create serious tensions in the rest of the family, which may in turn increase the baby's fussing.

Since colic seems to be an extension of fussing, it may be simpler to think of it as "heavy fussing." It's important to keep in mind that in almost all cases, no physical cause for the crying can be found; moreover, there is no reason to believe that the amount of crying puts the child at risk of any complication, or that somehow reducing the crying would help the baby in any physical way.

Frequently, fussy babies (particularly heavy fussers) don't just cry a lot; they have all kinds of extreme responses that make them generally more difficult to deal with. It seems that infants who cry excessively are also more sensitive, more irritable, and less easily soothed than average, and that they are more than usually active. Dr. Brazelton found further differences: for example, the lighter fussers tended to spend a lot more time sucking their fingers and pacifiers, whereas pacifiers didn't seem to placate the heavy fussers.

Could these heavy fussers be reacting to tension in their homes?
From his study of colicky babies with relaxed, experienced mothers, Dr. Brazelton concluded that heavy fussing did not necessarily indicate any neglect or abnormality in parenting.

It's more likely the other way around: the baby's constant fussing can put heavy stress on the parents, who then fall into reproaching themselves (or worse, each other) about their parenting abilities. Sometimes they refuse to give themselves a break and leave the baby with someone else. This guilty response is understandable but irrational, and it can only make matters worse; parents who find themselves slipping into it should discuss the problem with their physician.

Is it possible that the baby would fuss less if I responded differently?
In one three-group study, parents were given different instructions. The first group, the parents of 200 newborns, were given no special instructions. The second group, the parents of 70 newborns, were given the following instructions:

1. Try never to let your baby cry.

2. In working out the reason for his crying consider the following possibilities:

   a) The baby is hungry and wants to be fed.

   b) The baby is not hungry but wants to suck.

   c) The baby wants to be held and cuddled.

   d) The baby is bored and wants some stimulation—singing, smiling, talking, or play.

   e) The baby is tired and wants to sleep.

3. If the crying continues for more than five minutes of using one approach, then try another.

4. Work out your own way of exploring all the possibilities above.

The third group, the parents of another 70 newborns, were given baby slings and asked to carry their babies three more hours each day. All of these infants were monitored, using diaries, audio recordings, and questionnaires, and all the parents followed instructions, but no significant difference was found; regardless of the intervention, the infants fussed just as much.

In another study, it was found that if non-colicky babies were carried more, there was a 43 percent reduction in crying and fussing; however, it seems that colicky babies continue to cry, regardless of how much they are carried.

Since fussy babies often seem to be consoled by car motion, some parents assume that repetitive movements, vibrations, and "white noise" may do the same. But a study tested this by comparing three groups of fussy babies; parents in one group were given a device that vibrates the crib and makes a soft background noise, and those in another group were told to respond in the same way as the second group in the three-group study. The amount of fussing and the degree of parental stress improved with time, regardless of which group the families were in.

In short, no matter how much we try to soften the fussier babies' interaction with the environment, they cry just as much.

Colic: Looking for a Cause

Many factors have been suggested as reasons for colic—some external, such as parental stress, and some internal, such as digestive problems. But so far no theory has been convincingly supported by scientific studies.

 Could the colic be due to an allergy to cow's milk or soya milk?

An allergic reaction to cow's milk is a specific medical condition in which the baby's body reacts very adversely to even a small amount of the protein in cow's-milk formula, or to some of the cow's-milk protein that comes through from the mother's diet in her breast milk. It's also possible to be allergic to the soya protein in soya-milk formulas. People often confuse this specific allergy with *intolerance* for the sugar in milk, which is called "lactose"—a very different situation (see below). A true allergy is most unusual. If the baby did have a true allergy, there would be certain signs: he or she might be extremely colicky, and the colic would likely continue beyond the typical three-month mark. The baby might have diarrhea and vomiting and might not be gaining weight well. When the stool was tested, there might be traces of blood detected, even if they weren't visible to the naked eye.

A pediatric gastroenterologist who reviewed all the studies on this subject concluded that certain studies implicating cow's-milk protein as a cause of colic were looking at that very small percentage of extremely fussy infants who had symptoms of a true allergy to cow's-milk protein. There is no reason to assume that cow's milk also bothers non-allergic babies. Indeed, there is evidence that colic is *not* usually due to an allergy. For one thing, colic occurs equally in formula-fed and breast-fed babies.

Unless there are specific indications such as diarrhea and/or vomiting, poor weight gain, and/or traces of blood in the stool in an extremely colicky baby, a diagnosis of protein allergy should not be considered and the formula should not be changed.

 There seems to be so much gas in my baby's tummy. Could this be causing pain?

It's possible that all the crying and fussing result in the baby's swallowing a lot of extra air, and that this causes the gurgly tummy sounds and the excessive flatus (farting).

A number of studies have considered the possibility that colicky babies have lactose intolerance and are not completely digesting the lactose (sugar) present in breast milk or cow's milk. If this sugar is not completely digested, it passes into the lower part of the bowel; bacteria can feed on it there and produce gas. (For more information on lactose intolerance, see Chapter 12, "Feeding Your Child.")

A soya formula does not contain lactose, and there are cow's-milk formulas in which the lactose has been altered to be more digestible. Unfortunately, some studies show that when fussy babies are fed lactose-free milk, or an artificial lactase enzyme to help them digest lactose, they still cry and fuss just as much. It seems there is no scientific basis for using these formulas in an attempt to reduce the amount of gas.

 Could my baby be fussing because food isn't moving well in the intestine and the baby is getting cramps?

There is some evidence that babies who show high levels of motilin—the substance that controls the movement in the small intestine—may go on to develop symptoms of colic. But we do not yet have conclusive evidence of a connection, and in any case there is no proven treatment for the condition, even if it is related to colic.

Q Could my baby's spitting up be causing discomfort that looks like colic?

If the baby vomits, turns away from the breast or bottle, screams after the feeding starts, or wakes from sleep a few hours after feeding with heavy crying, and if these symptoms become worse when one would normally expect fussiness to subside (after age three months), consider the possibility that the baby is having bad heartburn. A trial of antacids is used in treating these babies.

Q If there's no physical problem, why does my baby cry so much?

The inconsolability is most likely part of the normal development of an infant who just a few months ago was in a completely different environment, not dependent on oral feeding or subject to changes in temperature, light, touch, etc. These infants are demonstrating their frustration with life outside the womb in the only way they can. Some infants seem to adjust very easily, whereas others struggle longer and harder. No parents, not even those with excellent responsiveness to their baby's needs, can recreate the coddled existence these babies may still recall.

Of course, we can't prove that this is the answer—yet it seems to be the only way to explain why these babies seem frustrated and angry as opposed to in pain; why studies searching for external causes produce inconclusive results (and studies on the issue of colic have filled pediatric literature for a long time); and why parents have such a difficult time settling these babies, even if they follow all the recommendations religiously.

Taking Care of a Fussy Baby

Desperate parents have tried any number of remedies to soothe their fussing babies. So far, no approach has been shown to be both safe and generally effective.

Q Might my baby fuss less if I stopped breast-feeding?

Formula-fed infants cry just as much as breast-fed ones, so there's no reason to switch to formula. Mothers often feel that they aren't producing enough milk, or that there must be something wrong with it, but this is not usually the case. Fussy babies are just harder to feed, by breast or formula; eventually they all get sufficient milk.

When 374 healthy infants were studied from birth to six weeks, it was found that infants who were switched from breast to formula did the same amount of fussing over a twenty-four-hour period as those who were consistently breast-fed. However, there was less evening crying in the formula-fed babies; crying tended to be spread through the day.

If your baby has a slow, rhythmical suckle, is having at least one substantial bowel movement each day from three weeks of age, and has at least six soaked diapers a day after the fifth day, the intake of milk is likely adequate.

Certain foods in the mother's diet are felt by some to affect the baby—these include apricots, beans, broccoli, cabbage, onions, peaches, prunes, rhubarb, and turnips. Although these foods don't cause fussing or crying, the general recommendation is that the suspected food be withdrawn from the diet for a week just to see if that makes any difference; if not, the food should be reintroduced. Remember that a nursing mother should have a healthy, well-balanced diet, and that excluding important foods may be harmful. (For more on breast-feeding and formulas, see Chapter 12, "Feeding Your Child.")

Would it help to change the formula?

Changing the formula generally makes no scientific sense. Parents often switch the type, brand, or preparation of their baby's formula for no logical reason. If any change is noted, it probably would have happened anyway.

Switching to a hydrolysed casein/whey formula (see Chapter 13) occasionally works. Babies who have heavy fussing that goes on for more than three months, a strong family history of allergic conditions like asthma or eczema, and symptoms like diarrhea, mucusy stools, vomiting, and/or microscopic amounts of blood in the stool (detected by a test done in your doctor's office) may have the rare allergy (mentioned above) to cow's-milk or soya protein. In these formulas the components have been broken down into smaller pieces that are less likely to cause allergic reactions. A hydrolysed casein/whey formula, which is generally a lot more expensive, should be used only on a trial basis. If it seems to work, that doesn't mean the baby is permanently allergic; the change may have been purely coincidental. Even true allergic reactions sometimes seem to disappear in a short time, so dairy and soya products should be reintroduced at a later date. It's important not to label your child "allergic" without cause.

Another experiment parents often try is introducing other foods, like cereal, on the grounds that the baby may be hungry. Formula actually contains more calories than cereal; moreover, cereal is often difficult to introduce into a baby's mouth at this age because he or she has not yet learned to accept a spoon. Studies have shown that infants introduced to cereals don't cry any less, although they seem to feed less often.

 What about all the advice people give me? Should I just ignore it?
Family, friends, and even professionals often assume that if a baby cries inconsolably, the parents must be doing something wrong. Their advice is copious, and frequently contradictory. The fact is that even first-time parents intuitively learn the best way to handle their baby, and endless input from other people is less than helpful. You may sometimes learn a useful specific tip from a book or a conversation, but don't feel obliged to try every new idea. There's a healthy balance between taking advice and having confidence in your own ability.

Remember that just because the baby is still fussing doesn't mean you've failed to provide everything. If all the baby's obvious needs have been met, it's not inappropriate to leave the child to cry. On the other hand, if you prefer to try to comfort the baby, that's fine too. Don't worry about spoiling the child at this point; you can work on establishing routines later, when you are past this stressful stage.

 Are there medicines or other remedies to treat fussing?
Medicines have been tested as treatments for colicky behavior. They fall into two categories: either they work but aren't safe, or they don't work but parents want to believe they do.

A good example of the latter is simethicone, which is supposed to work by making it easier for the baby to release swallowed gas. A recent study shows that a placebo (a look-alike syrup) works just as well. The same holds true for gripe water; a placebo was just as "effective." (Note that some formulations of gripe water contain alcohol.)

There are other medicines that make the baby sleepy. Examples include alcohol, diphenhydramine hydrochloride (Benadryl), chloral hydrate, and phenobarbital. Regardless of whether these medicines work or not, it is not acceptable for a parent to decide to use them on a baby.

In a study involving ninety-seven infants, the various ingredients of a prescribed colic mixture were tested individually against a placebo. The sedative ingredient, phenobarbital, worked no better than the placebo. Neither did the muscle relaxant, homatropine methylbromide—an atropine-like drug that relaxes the muscle in the bowel wall, and may also affect the baby's central nervous system. Neither did alcohol, which can cause convulsions in infants by making their level of blood sugar drop. Not only are these mixtures ineffective, but there have been reports of side-effects that were *acute life-threatening events* (ALTEs).

The one medicine that does improve fussy behavior—dicyclomine hydrochloride (Bentylol)—has also been associated with ALTEs, and is no longer used for this purpose.

Some parents are under the impression that herbal teas are safe, "natural" remedies for colic. In fact they may contain substances that work just like the atropine-related drug described above. Although one commercially pre-pared tea has been studied and may be effective, that doesn't mean that others are safe; poisonings with herbal teas are frequently reported.

In short, medication—pharmaceutical or herbal—is not a safe treatment for a fussing infant.

What if a colicky baby gets a real physical problem? How would I know?

Tell your doctor if you see signs of a milk or soya allergy, mentioned above, or if the baby has a fever.

If the baby is having hard and infrequent bowel movements, this suggests constipation (or holding back on bowel movements); your doctor can sug-gest ways to remedy that. If there are no bowel movements and the baby has any vomiting of a bright yellow or green color, this indicates a bowel block-age, a rare occurrence that requires immediate attention.

If you detect any specific part of the baby's body that seems tender, call your doctor immediately. Examples include pain when the diaper is changed; pain with hip movement, which could be a sign of infection of the hip joint; swelling and apparent tenderness in the groin, which could indi-cate a twist of the testis or a twisted hernia; or tenderness along any of the arms and legs or collar-bones, which might mean a broken bone.

Of course, it's impossible for you as a parent to know whether you are under- or overreacting. The best thing to do if you're in doubt is to have your doctor examine the baby and allay your concerns once and for all. Doctors are used to parents bringing their fussy babies back to the office week after week. They understand that a fussy baby can be very anxiety-provoking, and that knowing nothing is really wrong can provide a great deal of reassurance.

What can I do when I'm at my wits' end?

Being with a fussy baby day and night, losing more and more sleep, can make anyone exhausted and exasperated. It's essential to rely on family members and friends to give you a break. Some parents have difficulty leaving their baby, but resting up (and that means being away and out of earshot) enables you to return refreshed and better able to take good care of your baby.

Above all, recognize that at times this combination of weariness and desperation may result in a dangerous situation for both parent and child. It's important to express your feelings of frustration clearly to family members, friends, and your physician. Failing to do so can only make things worse for you. If you feel that you (or anyone else) might possibly lose control out of exasperation, *get help*. Never feel isolated; remember that there is always someone who can assist you. Parents who have recently moved to a new community can always call their local public health department and ask for the assistance of a health nurse, or look in the Yellow Pages for a medical doctor close by.

The Long-term Outlook

Parents often want to know if fussy babies are likely to have more difficult personalities and behavior when they grow up. Is a calmer baby likely to grow up to be more easygoing? The short answer seems to be that fussy behavior until about the age of three months (which is when most colicky babies settle down) is not associated with any long-term behavior problems. Calmer babies are just as likely to be challenging at a later stage as their fussier counterparts.

What if your infant is still inconsolable beyond the four-month mark? Studies show that these infants may go on to be more challenging children, but this is not a hard-and-fast rule.

Infants who remained very fussy beyond four months of age are often described by their parents as being very active children who just won't keep still. They are very alert and often don't seem happy in one position. Parents often pick them up and put them down repetitively in an attempt to make them more comfortable. Routines are often a problem; these babies tend to fight sleep, and as they get older they may be very resistant to eating. As well, they are more likely to develop constipation because they seem to resist having a bowel movement; in other words, they hold on too long. Stubbornness seems to be a hallmark of these children, and temper tantrums are more likely.

Whereas these infants initially appeared dissatisfied, later they seem to develop a pattern of provoking the hapless parent into situations of having to say no—at which point the child acts as if the parent is mean, and seems oblivious of the course of events that obviously led to this refusal. The child may pout and generally behave like a poor, mistreated, misunderstood little thing.

Families have to follow routines: bedtime means going to sleep at a specified time, certain items can't be touched because they are fragile or dangerous, siblings have to share. All of these realities may be misused by such children to force their parents to keep saying no. They seem unmoved by reasoning, and behavioral techniques are of limited value. The parents can only deal with the issue in a practical way, and realize that a stage has been reached where the environment can no longer bend to the whim of the child. Alas, we must wait and hope that the child eventually accepts this reality. There is only so much these parents can be expected to achieve, given the limited influences at their disposal. A reasonable and consistent approach and a healthy realization that this problem is not their fault is the best course we can suggest.

CHAPTER 5

Fever: When
Is It Serious?

● ●

Fever is one of the most common reasons for parents to take their child to see a doctor; it may account for a quarter of all doctor visits for children under two years of age. Unfortunately, although there have been many significant advances in our knowledge of fever, there are many things we still don't understand. Parents' fears about fever—sometimes referred to as "fever phobia," and perhaps made worse by the concern shown by many doctors—may lead to unnecessary phone calls and doctor visits, improper use of fever medications, and inappropriate attempts to bring down the child's temperature at all costs. Yet while parents worry so much about fever, many children are not particularly bothered by it.

What is fever, and what does it mean?

The first thing to remember is that fever is a symptom, not a disease. It helps us know that something unusual is going on in the child, and it may be the first sign that the child is unwell. It's the body's normal response to bacterial and viral infections and is a very common symptom in childhood illnesses.

Normally the temperature of the body ranges between 96.8°F and 100°F (36°C and 37.8°C). A fever is defined as a temperature above the normal range, which varies slightly, depending on where on the body it's measured. A temperature is considered a fever if it's above 99°F (37.2°C) under the arm, above 99.5°F (37.5°C) in the mouth, or above 100.4°F (38°C) measured rectally. The easiest place to take your child's temperature is under the arm; although it's not the most accurate measurement, that's probably not as important as simply knowing that the child does have a fever. For practical and safety reasons, children's temperatures should not be taken orally until they are over five years of age. Rectal temperatures are probably the most accurate, but the procedure may be frightening and uncomfortable for small children, and is often avoided these days.

Is fever in children helpful, harmful, or dangerous?

There is good information from laboratory studies supporting the view that fever is actually helpful, though some doctors still believe otherwise. The body protects itself against infections caused by germs, either bacteria or viruses, by a defense system known as the "immune response." This defense system is thought to be helped or "kick-started" by fever. Furthermore, the types of fever usually seen in children are not harmful; they do *not* cause brain damage or death. Although fever may cause convulsions (seizures) in some children (fewer than 5 percent), these convulsions are not harmful and have no long-term effects. Rare complications in children with fever are usually due to the underlying disease, such as meningitis, rather than the fever itself. Therefore, in trying to determine the seriousness of a fever, you should pay less attention to the height of the fever than to the child's behavior. Does he or she look sick and act sick? If not, the fever probably isn't serious.

Is your child sick?

In deciding whether your child is really sick, look for these features:

Well	*Sick*
lively and alert	droopy and apathetic
eating well	eating poorly
playing normally	ignoring toys
interested in surroundings	uninterested in surroundings
smiling at you	unresponsive
able to be comforted	inconsolable
normal color	pale/ashen complexion
moist mucous membranes (inside mouth, eyelids)	dry lips, no tears

Common Causes of Childhood Fever

The causes of fever vary, depending on the age of the child, and so does the seriousness of the fever.

What if my newborn baby has a fever?

In a child less than a month old, fever is often due to infection, sometimes bacterial and potentially serious. Dehydration (often the result of insufficient breast milk), overdressing, or an overheated environment may also cause a mild fever.

Any fever in this period requires immediate medical attention, not because of the fever itself, which is not dangerous, but because the underlying cause may be serious. Fever is often the only sign of infection in a newborn, who gives fewer warning signals of being unwell than does an older child. Other symptoms that may indicate serious illness in a newborn include a lower than normal temperature, not feeding properly, and spitting up feeds. It's particularly difficult to distinguish trivial problems from more serious illness at this age. Because of the dangers of bacterial infection, many doctors hospitalize infants less than a month old with fever, in order to observe them closely and start treatment with antibiotics while awaiting the results of lab tests. Treatment depends on how ill the baby looks, the results of blood tests, and other factors. If the lab tests are normal and the infant quickly returns to normal feeding, activity, and sleeping patterns, the hospital stay will be no longer than forty-eight hours.

What if my baby is between one and three months old?

In this case the fever is still worrisome, but much less so. Medical views about managing fever at this age are changing; your baby may be handled at home with very close observation and follow-up, or may be admitted to hospital, depending on the circumstances. Fever at this age is usually related to viral illness, but you should seek prompt medical attention if the infant is not lively, or is not behaving normally.

What about a baby over three months but under a year?

Fever in this age group is primarily the result of viral infections in the upper respiratory tract—in other words, the common cold. The infant characteristically has a runny nose with a clear discharge, stuffiness, and a cough or congestion; he or she may spit up or have the occasional loose bowel movement. The most common complication of a viral cold is an ear infection; you can often recognize this by the sudden development of irritability, crying, pulling of the ear, spitting up or vomiting, or not feeding well. (Teething around six months of age may produce many of these symptoms, but it's not associated with fever.) Often the clear discharge from the nose will become thicker and turn yellow or green, which may be a sign of a secondary bacterial infection.

A very high fever (as high as 105°F, or 40.5°C) that is not accompanied by other signs of sickness, except perhaps irritability, may indicate roseola, a common viral infection at this age (see Chapter 14, "Diseases and Medical Conditions"). Infants may also develop fever following immunization shots.

What about older children?

In children aged two to six, viral infections remain the most common cause of fever. Other possible causes at this age include strep throat, ear infections, bronchitis, and digestive- and urinary-tract infections.

In school-age children, viral respiratory-tract infections are the most common cause of fever. Strep throat and scarlet fever (strep throat with a rash) typically occur at this age. Urinary-tract infections, particularly in girls, may cause a fever as well. Bronchitis, pneumonia, and meningitis are uncommon causes of fever in school-age children.

When to get help

Any fever at all in a newborn infant should immediately be reported to a physician, or the baby should be taken to the nearest emergency department. Seek medical attention immediately for any child with a fever above 105°F (40.5°C) if the child is crying inconsolably, hard to awaken, or confused, or acts or looks very sick or has trouble breathing. Immediate medical aid should also be sought if the child has a stiff neck, has convulsions for the first time, or has purple spots (petechiae) anywhere on the skin. Children who have diseases such as leukemia or sickle cell anemia, or who are on immunosuppressants, should also have medical help immediately if they have any fever.

In children aged three months to two years, a fever above 101°F (38.5°C) for twenty-four hours merits a call to the doctor during regular office hours. A fever that continues for more than three days, irrespective of the age of the child, also demands a call to the doctor's office. Other reasons to seek medical help include a fever in association with behavioral changes such as crankiness or unusual quietness, or an appearance that makes you anxious.

Treating a Fever

The most important reason for treating a child who has a fever is to make the child more comfortable. In other words, the *child* should be treated, not the thermometer. A feverish child who is not uncomfortable requires no treatment, since the fever itself isn't dangerous.

Since most fevers are viral in origin, no treatment is available for the cause. However, if the fever has a bacterial cause such as an ear infection, your doctor can determine the appropriate medication to treat the infection.

What else can I do to make my child feel better?

All children with fever should be given extra fluids to prevent dehydration from sweating. They should be dressed in less clothing than usual, and where possible their activities should be reduced. If the child feels cold and is shivering with chills, which means the temperature is rising, a light blanket may give some immediate relief. Children should *not* be bundled up to "sweat out" the fever; this may be harmful as the body's excess heat can't escape. The room must not be overheated but rather kept at a comfortable 68°F (20°C). Children should not be covered with wet towels or sheets, which may make them uncomfortable, and alcohol sponging must never be used because the alcohol can be absorbed through the skin.

The use of lukewarm sponge baths is controversial; some studies indicate that these baths are no more effective than medication to lower the child's temperature, and in fact may make them uncomfortable with shivering and chills. (The use of sponge bathing has been abandoned in many busy emergency rooms.) Other physicians feel that a tepid bath does no harm and may be a useful technique for parents who are anxious to "do something." If you do decide to try a sponge bath, don't fill the tub too much; have the child sit in 8 inches (20 cm) of water, leaving most of the body exposed to help evaporation. If the sponging makes the child feel chilled, shivery, or unhappy, it should be stopped. For safety reasons, children should never be left alone in the bathtub.

Are there non-prescription drugs that bring down fever?

If medication is used to relieve the discomfort associated with a child's fever, acetaminophen is the drug of choice. It's not costly, it has few side-effects, and it's available in many forms for children, including drops, elixir (flavored syrup), flavored chewable tablets, capsules, caplets, and suppositories. Don't expect it to lower the child's temperature to normal, but it should bring it down to a more comfortable level. The dose range recommended is 10 to 15 mg/kg (milligrams per kilo of body weight) administered every four hours when necessary. (Thus a child who weighs 44 pounds, or 20 kilos, would be given a dosage of 200 to 300 mg.) It has been shown that many parents use a much lower dose of acetaminophen than the child's age or weight requires. It is perfectly safe and acceptable to use this drug at 15 mg/kg, and this dose is recommended by many doctors.

If the child vomits or spits up the medication immediately, or within ten to fifteen minutes, the entire dose may be given again. If the child can't tolerate the acetaminophen by mouth, a suppository can be tried.

Ibuprofen, another medication used to treat fever and pain, is currently *not approved* in Canada for children under twelve years of age. It's also not available in liquid form in Canada, though this form is used widely in the United States. The dose of ibuprofen is 5 to 10 mg/kg, given every six hours when needed. Side-effects are rare, but the drug has not been used for long enough in children for us to be certain of its absolute safety.

Remember that these medications are not cures, and should not be given automatically. If your feverish child is not uncomfortable, there is no need to bring the fever down.

A word about ASA and Aspirin

Acetylsalicylic acid is known generically as "aspirin" in the United States, but in Canada "Aspirin" is a brand name and the generic term is "ASA."

Although ASA is effective in reducing fevers, it is *not generally recommended* *for sick children* because of its side-effects. In particular, it's associated with Reye's syndrome, a rare condition that causes swelling of the brain and serious illness, and can be fatal.

Convulsions Due to Fever

Convulsions due to fever, or "febrile seizures," affect approximately one in twenty-five children who have a fever between the ages of six months and four to five years. The seizures are very upsetting, even terrifying, to parents, but they don't do any harm; the child won't die from the seizure and won't suffer any brain damage. Furthermore, studies show that 97 percent of all children with febrile seizures do not develop epilepsy, which is a different condition.

 What happens in a febrile seizure?

During the seizure the child loses consciousness and stiffens, the lips turn blue, and the whole body may begin to jerk. When the convulsive movements stop, the child regains consciousness but may be sleepy and groggy for a while. The most important thing is to remain calm and not panic, however frightening the convulsion may appear. Place the child on a soft surface, lying on his or her side. Don't put anything in the child's mouth. The child will *not* choke or "swallow" his or her tongue. The convulsion usually stops within a few minutes, without any medication. If it persists for more than five to ten minutes, take the child to the nearest doctor or hospital; convulsions that last longer than ten to twenty minutes may require medication to stop them. Calling an ambulance is safer than driving your child to a hospital at high speed when you are distracted by anxiety.

Children outgrow the tendency to have febrile seizures by the time they're four or five, but some children have recurrences. Even recurrent febrile seizures are not harmful and do not result in brain damage, death, or epilepsy. Unfortunately there is no known way of preventing the seizures. Although acetaminophen will lower the fever and make the child more comfortable, there is no evidence that it will prevent a seizure.

A child who has had a seizure associated with fever should be treated normally in all respects, and should resume normal activities. Being overprotective of a child just because there is a history of febrile seizures will only do harm.

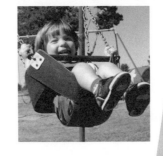

CHAPTER 6

Toilet Training

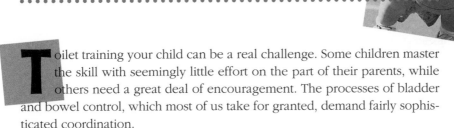

···

Toilet training your child can be a real challenge. Some children master the skill with seemingly little effort on the part of their parents, while others need a great deal of encouragement. The processes of bladder and bowel control, which most of us take for granted, demand fairly sophisticated coordination.

How do children learn to control their bladders?

Significant changes occur in bladder control from birth through childhood. In the infant, before bladder control is achieved, emptying and filling are automatic. The infant's bladder holds less than 2 ounces (about 50 ccs), so voiding cannot be delayed. Between the ages of one and two, as the brain matures, the infant becomes aware of the sensation of a full bladder and the need to urinate. In addition, bladder capacity increases so that the bladder doesn't have to empty as frequently. With further maturing, the child develops the ability to control the external sphincter muscle voluntarily, postponing urination until a toilet is available, even though the bladder is full. Daytime dryness is thus achieved.

How do children learn bowel control?

In infants, although the frequency and consistency of stool vary, depending on the diet, an individual pattern of stooling develops for each child and should not require parental intervention. Later, usually between two and three years of age, the child learns to recognize fullness of the lower large bowel as the sign that stooling is imminent, and to indicate that need. At first, this warning gives the parent a little time to supply a potty or toilet. Later, as

Bladder control

Two ureters carry urine from the kidneys to the bladder, a hollow structure surrounded by a muscular wall that relaxes when urine is being stored. When the muscle contracts, increasing the pressure in the bladder, and the bladder opening relaxes, the result is voiding of urine (urination). The urine then passes through the urethra and outside the body.

Two sphincters (muscular mechanisms) control the bladder. One is the inner sphincter at the bladder neck or outlet; stimulation of this muscle holds the urethra closed, keeping urine in the bladder, and relaxation allows voiding down the urethra. This mechanism is not under voluntary control. The other, the external sphincter, close to the outside end of the urethra, is under voluntary control. Stimulation of this muscle keeps the urethra closed and holds urine in the bladder; relaxation is essential for voiding.

Messages from the bladder to the brain (such as "I'm full!"), and from the brain to the bladder (such as "Hold on!") travel via the nerves of the spinal cord. These nerves are essential for the control of bladder function.

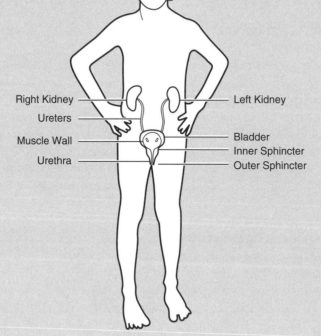

Right Kidney — Left Kidney
Ureters
Muscle Wall — Bladder
Urethra — Inner Sphincter
— Outer Sphincter

the child gains more control over the external sphincter of the bowel, stooling can be delayed. But while a delay may be convenient, note that repeated or prolonged withholding can lead to problems with constipation, stretching and thinning of the bowel muscles, and even soiling (see below). A child who "needs to poo" should be given the chance as soon as possible.

By the time they start to recognize that stooling is imminent, most children have already stopped stooling into diapers at night. Daytime bladder control is usually achieved next, followed by daytime bowel control.

Bowel control

The nutrients from our food are absorbed into the bloodstream from the part of the bowel called the small intestine. After passing through this part of the bowel, any remaining contents enter the large intestine, which is responsible for further absorption of water and formation of the final stool. The wall of the large intestine is composed of muscle fibers and nerves. The muscle propels the waste products towards the anal opening, and the nerves carry messages between the muscle and the brain.

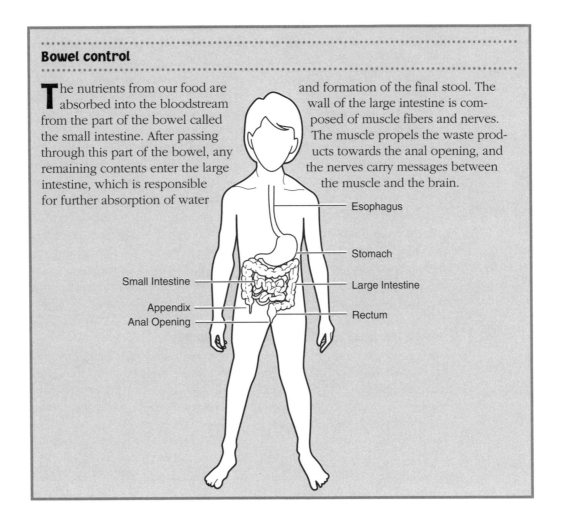

Esophagus

Stomach

Small Intestine

Large Intestine

Appendix

Rectum

Anal Opening

How will I know when my child is ready for toilet training?

Children need to be ready both physically and temperamentally for this important event. Although it's possible to predict the reflex emptying of an infant's bladder or bowel, and therefore to be lucky enough to catch the urine or stool in a vessel, this is not the same as the infant mastering bladder and bowel control. In deciding when to begin real toilet training, you should consider several factors.

Often children begin to imitate siblings or parents, and to show an interest in the passage of urine and stool from their bodies and the use of potties or toilets. Signals that the child is aware of a full bladder or bowel may be facial expressions, wriggling movements, or other signs that parents usually interpret quickly and correctly. This is an important first step in toilet training. The bladder should have matured to the point that your child is able to stay dry for several hours and pass a reasonable quantity of urine at each voiding. The desire for independence and increasing competence will lead your child to an interest in managing toiletting, and allowing the child to progress at his or her own pace, without conflict and tension, is thought to be important.

It's reasonable to start training when your child is able to walk, to get to the potty or toilet without help. The combination of understanding the purpose of the toilet, being aware of the need to urinate or stool, and feeling displeasure at being wet or dirty is important in the process. If these milestones coincide with the child's desire to please you by mastering the skills *before* the child reaches the phase of saying no to everything, toilet training can often be easily achieved. Consequently you should try to be sensitive to your child's development, provide opportunities for mastering toiletting skills without coercion, and postpone the process if the child shows resistance.

What's the best approach to toilet training?

There's a wide variety of cultural influences on toilet-training methods, and your family and cultural expectations should be respected and integrated into your method of toilet training, and indeed into all aspects of child-rearing. There are no good studies to tell us which method of toilet training is the most successful. However, some suggestions have been accepted as "good advice."

The use of a potty as an introduction to the toilet is favored by many. The potty has the advantages of being a more appropriate size for a young child, being closer to the floor, and allowing the child's feet to remain on the floor; it's also portable. Some children express a fear of the toilet, imagining that monsters will "nip their bottoms" or that they'll fall in and be flushed away. This fear can be minimized by simple reassurance and by providing adaptable seating and a bench under the feet. Appropriate posture, with the hips and knees at right angles and the feet against a firm surface, may make defecation easier. Be sure to allow the child enough time for complete urination or defecation, and to encourage successful completion, as this will build up the child's sense of accomplishment.

Young children need help in using the toilet for a while, but as they get better at dressing and undressing they learn to manage visits on their own. Accidents may still occur in the daytime, as a child can delay urination only a few minutes after feeling the initial urge. As the child matures, these accidents become less frequent. If a child at any time becomes difficult to handle or resists toileting regularly, it's usually better to stop your efforts for a few months and then start again. Children usually learn quickly when they are ready.

What about nighttime?

Bowel emptying at night has usually stopped before daytime bowel training begins. However, night wetting usually persists after daytime dryness has been achieved. There is no clear evidence whether the method and timing of toilet training accelerate or retard nighttime dryness. When your child has achieved reasonable control in the day, the diapers can be left off except at night. When he or she is dry on wakening, nighttime dryness has been achieved and the diapers can be abandoned.

What about children who keep on wetting?

Most normal children achieve daytime dryness by age four and nighttime dryness by age five, though boys tend to be later than girls. Persistence of wetting beyond these ages is referred to as "daytime (diurnal) enuresis" and "nighttime (nocturnal) enuresis"—also known as "bed-wetting." Daytime and nighttime wetting may both be present. If the child has been dry for a minimum of six months and then has an onset of wetting, day or night, it's called "secondary." If such a dry period has never occurred, the wetting is "primary."

Daytime wetting occurs in about 1 percent of children aged seven to twelve. But 15 percent of children are still wetting the bed at night at age five. As they mature, some of them outgrow the problem; only 5 percent of ten-year-olds, 2 percent of sixteen-year-olds, and fewer than 1 percent of adults have this problem. The factors that contribute to nighttime wetting beyond the age of five are a delay in the maturing of the mechanisms required for bladder control, and an inherited predisposition. If both parents were bed-wetters, there is a 77 percent chance of their child being a bed-wetter. If one parent was a bed-wetter, there is a 44 percent chance.

Your child's mastery of bladder control should be discussed at your regular visits to the child's physician. You can express your concerns about any delays, and seek advice on maintaining a reasonable plan for toilet training. If unusual urinary symptoms develop, such as frequency of urination or pain on urination, arrange for assessment by a physician. Persistence of wetting beyond the expected age should also trigger a further assessment.

How will the doctor make this assessment?

The doctor will take a history of many aspects of the child's problem. It will be important to know whether the accidents are happening in the daytime or nighttime, or both, and whether the wetting is primary or secondary. The doctor will ask if there are any associated symptoms, such as pain on urination, that might suggest a urinary-tract infection. A history of the child's toilet training is helpful in understanding daytime difficulties in particular, while a history of the child's general health and development lets the doctor consider any other medical or developmental problems that might explain the delay in bladder control. The doctor may also ask if you are concerned about any other behavioral problems that might reflect the maturity or compliance of the child, or any fears the child may have. For example, fear of the dark can make it difficult for a child to leave bed at night to go to the bathroom. It's also helpful to know what treatments have been tried so far.

A family history, particularly of the parents, is useful to determine if either parent was a bedwetter. If there is any family history of kidney disease, you may be anxious to rule out the possibility of kidney disease in your child.

The doctor will also explore the emotional aspects of the wetting. How does the child cope? How is the child's self-esteem? What does the wetting prevent the child from doing? For example, does he or she miss sleepovers with friends, or going to camp? What is the attitude of the family towards the bed-wetting? Is either parent upset, angry, or frustrated? How have the parents responded to each bed-wetting episode? Do they blame the child, or each other?

The doctor will then do a full examination, with particular attention to the abdomen, the spine, the genitalia, and the nerves that supply the organs that control urination.

For children who have nighttime wetting as their only problem, a urine test is usually enough to rule out urine problems. If the child has daytime wetting, a urine test will still be appropriate, but it may be necessary to do other tests as well, depending on what the doctor finds.

Why do some children have "accidents" after they are toilet trained?

The child may be too busy playing to answer the body's signals that the bladder is full, or may have suppressed the urge on several occasions, until the need to urinate became overwhelming and the child couldn't make it to the bathroom in time. It's important to watch for signals of your child's desire to urinate, and especially for signals that he or she is trying to suppress the urge—for example, squatting, pressing a heel into the genital area, dancing around, or crossing the legs. You should encourage your child to empty his or her bladder when the "need to go" signal occurs; that habit plays an important role in the mastery of urinary habits.

Sometimes stress is involved; the hospitalization of a young child, separation from parents, or a family break-up may make a child regress to wetting. The recurrence of daytime wetting may also signal the onset of a medical problem such as a urinary-tract infection, so a physician's advice should be sought. Other symptoms of urinary-tract infections may include frequency of urination, altered smell and colour of the urine, and possibly fever and lower-abdominal pain. A urine test will be required to rule out the possibility of infection. Once the problem has been dealt with, retraining in toilet habits may be required.

Why do some children keep on bed-wetting?

Parents often note that their bed-wetting child is a deep sleeper. Sleep studies have failed to show that bed-wetting is associated with a particular stage of sleep; however, there is some evidence that arousal times are different for bed-wetters than for children who have nighttime control of urination. Perhaps it just takes these children too long to wake up. There is no evidence that small bladder capacity, serious psychological disorder, or allergic problems are responsible for most cases of bed-wetting. Physical abnormalities occasionally cause the persistence or onset of nighttime wetting beyond five years of age, but that possibility can be checked by the physician.

What can I do about a bedwetter?

You can start by explaining the likely cause of the problem to your child, clearly and in age-appropriate language. In most cases this means explaining that the tendency is inherited and developmental, and outside the child's control, and that it's not any kind of illness. Have an open discussion of other causes the child may have heard you blame, and reassure him or her that no one thinks the problem is rooted in laziness.

As for practical measures, once it's clear that the child has no underlying kidney problems, supportive measures should be adopted. Some families choose to live with the problem, and manage it by using plastic sheets on the bed and changing the sheets immediately after a wetting episode, or in the morning if the child has not awakened. There are mattress covers available that absorb the majority of the wetness and can be placed immediately underneath where the child sleeps. Sometimes children are encouraged to participate in stripping the bed; this is appropriate as long as it's done to encourage self-sufficiency, and not in a punitive fashion. Some parents say that encouraging the child to wear pull-up diapers of an appropriate size is helpful. Most children over the age of six find this babyish and unacceptable, but the strategy may be useful for overnight trips. The child can often manage such diapers on his or her own, if easy disposal is available; failing that, send along a plastic bag to ensure safe transportation home.

A few children develop skin irritation and rashes secondary to the wetness, but the vast majority do not. If a rash does develop, changing the wet clothing as soon as urination occurs is an important preventive measure, and barrier creams will help prevent the rash from getting worse.

Would it help if I limited my child's fluid intake after supper?

This simple maneuver is successful in some children, but certainly not in all. It makes sense that drinking large quantities of liquid before bedtime will challenge any bladder during the night hours. However, normal amounts of fluid should be allowed and no child should be made to go to bed thirsty.

What about waking the child up for a bathroom trip before I go to bed myself?

Some parents find that rousing the child to go to the bathroom at their bedtime prevents further wetting during the night. However, many children don't wake up enough at this time to make themselves urinate. If the strategy works for your child, by all means use it. However, it is not appropriate to disturb your own night's sleep with repeated awakenings to rouse the child.

Should I try some sort of reward system?

You might try putting up a big calendar and letting your child keep a record of dry nights and wet nights. A dry night earns the child a sticker or gold star, and some further reward if you want. This method of rewarding dry nights has been shown to be successful in approximately 20 percent of children, so it's worth trying as a first-line measure. Unfortunately, some children relapse and are unable to maintain dryness in spite of the rewards.

Do bed-wetting alarms work?

The most commonly used bed-wetting alarm consists of a battery-operated machine; a device for sensing wetness, which is attached to the child's underwear or pyjamas, close to the urethral opening; and a buzzer attached to the child's clothing on the shoulder, close to the ear. The first few drops of urine passed should touch the sensor and set off the alarm, which should waken the child, and thus stop the urination. The child then disconnects the alarm and gets up to go to the bathroom. If the child has more than one wet episode in a night, the underwear should be changed and the alarm reset to catch the next bed-wetting episode. This method is the most successful form of treatment available and works for 70 to 90 percent of children. However, the child must be mature enough, developmentally and emotionally, and motivated enough to deal with the signals. Although you can come and attempt to assist the child in waking up, perhaps by placing a wet cloth on his or her forehead, it's essentially the child who must respond to the alarm. As this is a training regimen, be prepared to try the alarm for at least a month, and probably two. Although 20 percent of children relapse when they stop using the alarm, the majority remain dry.

The alarm system is less likely to work for a child of six or seven, and more likely to work for the child of nine or older, particularly one who is very highly motivated to achieve dryness. A calendar is kept during the period of treatment to record wet and dry nights, as well as "damp only" episodes when the alarm roused the child enough to pass most of the urine in the toilet. It's interesting that children who achieve dryness from this treatment don't necessarily wake up at night to pass their urine, but are able to sleep through the night. Presumably their bodies learn to hold urine in spite of the bladder being full. The alarm systems cost around $50 and have replaceable batteries. Of course, they don't work for deaf children, and they may not be suitable for children who sleep with siblings or parents, or those who are too fearful of the noise to use the alarm successfully.

There are older alarm systems that are placed under the bedsheets, but they are less successful as more urine needs to be passed before the alarm goes off. There is also a system that delivers an electric shock when the child wets. However, this is not recommended for younger children. If a teenager who is resistant to all other forms of therapy wants to try this type of alarm, some physicians support its use. Take care that the contact of the electrodes with the skin doesn't cause skin irritation. A new alarm with a vibrating signal has recently become available, but there are as yet no studies to document its effectiveness.

Q I've heard of something called "Azrin's system"—what's that?

This multidimensional approach to bed-wetting uses several techniques to reinforce dryness, including nighttime wakening, positive and negative reinforcement, bladder-control training, and the use of a urine alarm. The alarm is a proven form of therapy, but the addition of the other components has not clearly been shown to be useful.

Q Do bladder-control exercises do any good?

Some (not all) children with bed-wetting may have a smaller functional bladder capacity than normal for their age. Bladder-training exercises have been attempted, to encourage children to hold urine a few minutes beyond their initial urge to urinate. Studies are inconclusive as to whether these exercises make a difference to the frequency of bed-wetting.

Q Aren't there any medications that help?

Several medications have been shown to be of benefit in treating bed-wetting. However, it's essential to look at the harm a medication may do, as well as its success, since bed-wetting is a developmental condition that will eventually go away on its own.

Imipramine (Tofranil) was originally introduced as an antidepressant but was found to be successful in reducing bed-wetting episodes. It's effective in only about half the children who try it, and its side-effects include emotional instability, sleep disturbances, lethargy, dry mouth, and mild stomach upsets, to name a few. However, many children tolerate the medicine without any difficulty. Note that imipramine is a *very dangerous drug* when too much is taken; overdoses can lead to heart and breathing problems, convulsions, and even death. Be sure to keep it locked away from children, except for the prescribed dose.

More recently, desmopressin acetate (DDAVP) has been introduced for the treatment of bed-wetting. This is a different form of a naturally occurring substance called "antidiuretic hormone," which helps the body retain water and prevents its excretion. It has been suggested that bed-wetting children suffer from decreased levels of antidiuretic hormone, or do not respond normally to it. Although this has not been proven conclusively, DDAVP decreases bed-wetting in approximately half of children. It is administered by nasal spray, in a dosage of one to four puffs (10 to 40 micrograms), before going to bed. It may not work if the child has a cold or allergic nasal inflammation, as this can interfere with its absorption. Its side-effects include irritation of the nose and eyes, but it is usually well tolerated. It does have a very low risk of causing significant disturbances in the body's fluid and salt composition, which can lead to convulsions, so whenever the child is sick with vomiting and diarrhea the drug should be discontinued. Also, caution the child against drinking unnecessary excess fluid while on the medication. DDAVP can be very useful for ensuring dryness on overnight stays with friends or during attendance at camp. The benefit usually ceases when the medication is stopped.

Oxybutynin (Ditropan) has not been proven useful in nighttime wetting, but has been used successfully to help improve bladder capacity in some children with daytime wetting.

What about non-drug therapies?

Some parents have found hypnotherapy helpful in getting their children to stop bed-wetting. However, this remains a controversial area and there is no clear evidence to support its use.

Rarely, emotional disturbances are involved in bed-wetting. In such cases, psychotherapy may help; stresses can be discussed, and appropriate support mechanisms put in place. However, there is no role for psychotherapy in the treatment of most bed-wetting children.

What about a child who defecates in the wrong place?

This is called "soiling"—the repeated voluntary or involuntary passage of stools in inappropriate places, such as into underwear or onto the floor. Most children have achieved bowel control by age four if they have otherwise normal development. Persistence of soiling beyond that age is referred to as "primary" soiling, or encopresis. If the child has had a minimum of six months without soiling and then begins to soil, this is called "secondary" encopresis. Unfortunately, soiling leaves an offensive odour, so the child may be ridiculed and isolated. There is often friction within the family, and the child may be the target of anger and blame.

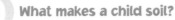 **What makes a child soil?**

The most common cause is constipation. Retention of stools leads to stretching of the large bowel wall, which leads to a decrease in its ability to contract and propel the contents forward. More water is absorbed from the stool because it stays longer in the large bowel, and so larger and harder stools are formed. The passage of these stools is often painful, and may even cause stretching and tearing of the anal opening (fissures); as a result, the child may delay stooling, which makes the problem even worse. There are also some children who have incomplete emptying of the bowel; they seem to have "regular" bowel movements but in fact retain considerable amounts of stool. In either case, the retained stool can form "rocks," and then softer stool may leak around these, resulting in soiling.

Several factors are believed to contribute to the development of this problem. In infancy, constipation, abnormalities of the lower bowel (anus and rectum), and forceful interventions by parents may set the scene for later development of soiling. In the toddler and preschool years, painful or difficult stooling (for a variety of reasons), forceful toilet training, psychosocial stresses that interfere with toilet training, or unusual fear of the toilet may contribute further to the risk. As the child passes into school age, other risk factors emerge: avoidance of school toilets, difficulties with staying at tasks (attention deficit), busy family lifestyles, and similar psychosocial stresses. Many children cope with these stresses, but some, especially those with several risk factors, go on to develop soiling.

Constipation is not always involved; diarrhea may also lead to loss of control over stool. Acute infections or gastroenteritis in a young child may result in temporary soiling. However, this usually resolves itself. Repeated episodes of loose stool that can't be traced to underlying medical problems are probably more akin to "irritable bowel syndrome" in adults.

There is also a small group of children who have "manipulative" soiling, which is not caused by constipation, though constipation may be present. These children appear to be expressing strong feelings (anger or sadness) through their bowels.

Rarely, a medical problem lies behind the soiling.

What can I do if my child is soiling?

It's very important to get a full medical assessment: a history of bowel habits, toilet training, other developmental and health issues, family history, and stresses on the child, followed by a complete physical examination. Special tests are occasionally done to clarify or rule out medical causes for the problem.

The treatment will depend on the cause or the factors contributing to the soiling. Any constipation can be managed by a regimen of altered diet and improved bowel habits, to empty the bowel of retained stool and encourage the passage of smaller, softer stools. Stool softeners or other laxatives may also be recommended. Careful attention to regular toilet visits, provision of adequate time for stooling, and rewarding of appropriate stooling behavior are critical. If serious underlying stresses or problems exist, more specific therapy will be required.

CHAPTER 7

Spitting Up, Vomiting, and Diarrhea

· ·

Spitting up and regurgitation often occur in early infancy, and are usually related to feeding. The difference between spitting up, regurgitation, and vomiting is often not clear, and these symptoms may seem to merge into one another at times. Many infants have them to varying degrees in the first few months of life.

Q **What's the difference between "spitting up" and "regurgitation"?**

Many babies voluntarily expel milk while they're feeding, pushing the liquid out of their mouths with their tongues. The amount of breast milk or formula lost this way is small, and simple "spitting up" by itself is never associated with significant disease unless an infant fails to gain weight and thrive. At times babies spit up simply because they've taken in too much milk, or because a bubble of air is escaping the stomach.

Spitting up is not a good reason to change a child's formula. It's a benign condition that usually improves by six months of age and resolves itself by eight to twelve months of age.

Regurgitation is also common in early infancy, but it can be an indication of serious gastrointestinal illness at this age. Regurgitation is the effortless expulsion of the contents of the stomach; the amount of regurgitated food varies and may or may not be significant. This symptom may occur at any time, with the infant in any position, but it's most common immediately after the child has eaten. Usually liquid and solid foods are regurgitated equally. If regurgitation persists, it should be evaluated by your child's physician, who will want to know how soon after birth you noticed the baby regurgitating, and whether it makes a difference how the baby is positioned after feeding. Most important, the doctor will check whether your child has gained enough weight since the regurgitation began. If the weight gain has been normal, there is likely very little to be concerned about, but the symptom needs to be observed. The doctor will also want to know if the child is choking during the episodes of regurgitation, and if the child's lips turn blue or he or she seems to stop breathing momentarily. These symptoms are more serious indications of illness. There are several gastrointestinal conditions associated with persistent regurgitation in childhood, but the most common is gastroesophageal reflux (GER). Premature infants are very likely to have GER.

 What exactly is GER?

In GER, the valve at the lower end of the esophagus, leading to the stomach, is not as tight as normal. In the first eight to twelve weeks of life, all children have some looseness of this valve. Between three and nine months of age, the valve tightens and the reflux (regurgitation) becomes less frequent. No treatment is necessary unless the episodes of reflux are accompanied by "blue spells"—episodes where breathing seems temporarily stopped—or the infant is not gaining weight. In a more severely affected infant, repositioning the child after feeding, changing feeding routines, and thickening the feeds may reduce the reflux.

Persistent severe GER may be associated with weight loss and chronic irritability. The irritability is the result of stomach acid and partially digested food flowing back into the lower esophagus. In extreme cases the irritation causes bleeding, and anemia may result. If the situation continues unchecked for a long time, the lower esophagus may narrow and require surgical treatment. Severe GER can also be responsible for recurrent coughing and wheezing episodes in infancy, due to stomach contents entering the back of the throat and the lungs.

 Can allergies cause regurgitation?

In past years, regurgitation has been blamed on a child's allergy to cow's milk or to other foods. Many infants are changed from cow's-milk formula to soy-milk formula to relieve the problem. Although some seem to improve after the change, most do not, and in those who do the difference may be coincidental. Today most doctors do not associate the symptom of regurgitation alone with milk or food allergy. However, if an infant has a history of chronic sniffles or a clear nasal discharge that defies explanation, has other allergic reactions such as eczema, or has a strong family background of food allergy, then allergy may be considered as a cause.

What's the difference between regurgitation and vomiting?

Vomiting is the *forceful* expulsion of stomach contents. It's a more serious symptom than spitting up or regurgitation, and can lead to significant medical problems if it persists. In older children who don't appear severely ill, vomiting may disappear without treatment within twelve to twenty-four hours, but a young infant or child who is vomiting needs to be assessed sooner because of the risk of dehydration. Vomiting can be associated with minor illnesses, but it can also be the first symptom of more serious problems, such as intestinal obstruction, inflammation, or meningitis. That's why it's important to tell the doctor when a young child—especially an infant—is vomiting.

That doesn't mean that all vomiting is serious. A child who is suddenly frightened may vomit, as may a child who is angry, upset, or just very excited. Sometimes children vomit simply because they've gobbled up too much of a favourite food.

When you report vomiting to your child's doctor, you can help by having an accurate description of your child's condition in your mind. Does the child appear unwell? How long has the symptom been present? Is there a fever? If so, how high is it? Are there symptoms such as headache, neck pain, abdominal pain, diarrhea, rash, earache, cough, or sore throat? Is the child producing urine in the usual amount? Is the material being vomited bile-stained (greenish) or blood-tinged? Can the child keep down *any* food or fluid? Do specific foods seem to cause the problem? Has the child taken any medication that might provoke vomiting as a side-effect, or come in contact with spoiled food? Is anyone else in the house ill? Could the child have accidentally got into any medication or household products? From the answers to these questions your doctor can decide whether the child can be managed at home, needs to be seen in the office, or needs prompt referral to your local emergency department.

When vomiting needs immediate attention

A child with bile-stained or bloody vomitus, who is vomiting frequently and has a distended, swollen abdomen and severe abdominal pain accompanied by lethargy and irritability, is in urgent need of medical attention. A young child who has been vomiting longer than twelve to twenty-four hours, is unable to hold down any fluids, and has reduced urinary output should be assessed by a doctor.

What are the more serious causes of vomiting?

In the period shortly after birth, vomiting can be due to obstruction of the gastrointestinal tract. The most common reason for this is a muscular obstruction to the outflow valve of the stomach, called "pyloric stenosis." The condition is typically seen in newborns about five to six weeks of age, but may begin as early as two to four weeks of age. The vomiting is very forceful (projectile) and worsens as time goes on. The condition is more common in boys than in girls, and tends to run in families.

Infection of the urinary tract and *meningitis* are two serious conditions that may first appear as vomiting in early infancy. Meningitis is an uncommon condition caused by bacteria inflaming the tissues around the brain (meninges). It is associated with fever, headache, neck stiffness, and extreme irritability. If not diagnosed and treated early, it leads to drowsiness, coma, and possible permanent brain damage or death. Significant fever along with vomiting in an infant who is feeding poorly and appears unwell should alert you to these possibilities.

Gastroesophageal reflux (GER) is an important cause of vomiting in an infant, as noted above. Infants who have severe GER may regurgitate their food and vomit as well. In severely affected infants, the vomiting may be blood-tinged. Typically, such infants are poor eaters and fail to thrive.

Celiac disease is a rare condition caused by an inborn inability of the intestinal lining to handle gluten, a protein found in wheat. The resultant inflammation causes diarrhea and the inability of the intestine to absorb necessary nutrients. What usually brings these children to the doctor is chronic diarrhea and poor weight gain. Children with celiac disease who are given a gluten-free diet do extremely well.

Rumination, the regurgitation of both liquid and solid food in a purposeful manner, can occur during feedings but is more common after a meal is completed. It can occur in any situation but is more common in children who are mentally handicapped or have significant mental illness. GER can be associated with rumination.

Intestinal infection is another common cause of vomiting in infants and toddlers. Usually fever and diarrhea are also present. Viral infections account for the vast majority of these illnesses, but about 20 per cent are caused by bacterial infections. Often the stool contains blood. The high fever associated with these infections may lead to a febrile convulsion.

Intussusception is a serious but uncommon problem that occurs in infants and toddlers, in which one section of intestine "folds" inside another. The onset of attacks of severe abdominal pain in a previously healthy child, accompanied by vomiting and the eventual appearance (in most cases) of a red jelly-like stool (blood), suggests this condition. Early diagnosis of intussusception leads to successful treatment. Fortunately, the other causes of intestinal obstruction in childhood are quite rare.

Inflammation of the appendix is the commonest reason for abdominal surgery in childhood. Although abdominal pain is the main symptom, vomiting commonly accompanies the pain. This condition is unusual in infants and toddlers; it's much more likely to occur in older children and adolescents. The appendix, a small piece of intestine that serves no useful role, may get obstructed and inflamed. Abdominal pain and fever, with vomiting and no diarrhea, should prompt you to have your child checked for appendicitis. If your child has this problem, surgery to remove the inflamed appendix is necessary and solves the problem forever.

Neurological conditions can also cause vomiting in children. A head injury, with or without loss of consciousness, must be monitored closely if the child begins to vomit. Migraine headaches can also be accompanied by vomiting. Although brain tumors are infrequent in childhood, the presence of a persistent headache accompanied by vomiting in a child who does not feel nauseated and does not have a fever must be brought to the attention of the child's physician.

Vomiting may also be associated with heavy bouts of coughing. For example, whooping cough is frequently associated with vomiting, and so is asthma.

Q How can I stop my child's vomiting?

Fortunately, most children stop vomiting without any medical treatment. It's important to position a vomiting child on his or her side so that vomited material won't be breathed into the lungs. Children who vomit continuously and are unable to keep any liquids down, or who have diarrhea and fever, must be watched closely for dehydration.

Q Are there medications that stop vomiting?

It's extremely important *not* to use over-the-counter remedies for childhood vomiting without consulting your doctor. Some medications can mask a child's symptoms, or prevent you from making an accurate assessment of your child's progress. Few, if any, of these remedies are truly effective in controlling the cause of vomiting.

The risks of dehydration

When the body loses large quantities of water, through vomiting, diarrhea, or even just sweating, it also loses essential minerals called "electrolytes." Without enough water and electrolytes, the body's functioning can be seriously impaired. Dehydration is potentially life-threatening, and requires early recognition and treatment.

Dehydration can be recognized by lack of moisture in mucous membranes; look for a dry mouth, no saliva production, an absence of tears, weight loss, lethargy and irritability, and decreased urine output. The urine may be abnormally dark in color, because waste products are less diluted with water.

Dehydration can be treated by restoring the lost fluids and electrolytes. Studies have shown that early use of an oral electrolyte solution (such as Pedialyte, Lytren, or Infalyte) is the best treatment.

If a child has been vomiting, it's a good idea to wait an hour after the last episode before attempting rehydration. Then give a small volume of oral electrolyte solution—60 to 90 ml (2 or 3 ounces)—every thirty to forty minutes, until the child seems stable enough to accept plain foods. Occasionally, children who don't respond to oral electrolyte solution need to be hospitalized and given intravenous fluids.

If the child is dehydrated, use an oral electrolyte solution to combat the dehydration. Once the child has kept down the solution for several hours without significant vomiting, simple solids—bread, crackers, pasta, potatoes—can be reintroduced into the diet. A breast-feeding infant can have breast milk. If these foods are well tolerated, the child can return to a normal diet with formula or milk in thirty-six to forty-eight hours. A child who can't hold down oral replacement fluids or simple solid foods in the first twelve to twenty-four hours should be assessed by a doctor.

Diarrhea

The normal pattern of bowel movements varies in consistency and frequency, depending on the child's age and the composition of the diet. In the newborn period, babies who are breast-fed may have up to ten small bowel movements per day, often one after each feeding. The normal stool of a breast-fed infant has a pasty consistency and a mustard-like color. By the end of the twelfth week, the frequency of the infant's stool has decreased. Some infants begin to have semifirm stool once daily or every other day. By the age of eighteen to thirty months, most children have one or two formed bowel movements each day.

As a parent, you become accustomed to the consistency, amount, and frequency of your infant's bowel movements. Suddenly they may become loose, and increase in volume and frequency. The color may change, and a foul odor may be evident when the stools are passed. This is diarrhea.

Is diarrhea serious?

An occasional loose stool is no cause for alarm. Most often, diarrhea is mild and clears up without treatment in one or two days. However, if the symptom is accompanied by high fever, if your child appears ill, and if he or she has copious quantities of explosive movements, with or without vomiting, consult the doctor.

Diarrhea or loose bowel movements can be caused by simple overfeeding. In this case the stools are semiformed and can be frequent, but are seldom discolored or malodorous. A child should never be forced to take more milk than he or she seems to want.

Many parents of young toddlers are concerned by the presence of undigested food particles in the child's loose stool. This finding is not abnormal, and means little in terms of diagnosis.

The sudden onset of loose, watery bowel movements along with increased stool volume may be a more serious sign, especially if the child is vomiting and feverish. Severe diarrhea, especially in young infants, merits a call to the doctor, as well as close observation of the child because of the risk of dehydration.

What else causes diarrhea?

Diarrhea can be a side-effect of medication, especially certain antibiotics. If your child has unexpected diarrhea and is taking medications, check with your doctor or pharmacist.

When a breast-fed infant develops diarrhea, the mother may continue to breast-feed as long as the child's symptoms remain mild. If the infant is otherwise well, look for recent changes in the mother's diet, or any new medication the mother may be taking; either one may possibly be affecting the baby. Other noninfectious causes of diarrhea include acute poisoning with iron, lead, mercury, or fluoride; food poisoning; and intussusception (see above).

When the lining of a child's intestine is damaged because of infection, diarrhea is the result. The damaged lining can no longer digest or absorb foods normally, and the lack of complete digestion and absorption is complicated by the fact that the damaged bowel lining can secrete minerals and fluid into the intestine. Until recently, feeding the child liquids flavored with large amounts of sugar was a common recommendation. In fact this can make diarrhea *worse*; the build-up of unabsorbed sugar may cause the body to secrete more water into the intestine, making the stools even more watery.

"Enteritis" is inflammation or damage of the intestinal wall. When the lining of the stomach is also inflamed or damaged, the condition is called "gastroenteritis." In children, the commonest cause of acute diarrhea is enteritis brought on by a virus. Fever may be present, as may vomiting. The bowel movements of children with viral gastroenteritis are greenish and very liquid. On occasion it may be difficult to distinguish them from urine in the diaper. If the stools look bloody or are black in appearance, there may be bleeding from the bowel lining. Blood in the stools can be associated with viral diarrhea, but more commonly indicates bacterial enteritis. In any case, bloody stools should be reported to a doctor. Bacterial enteritis may also be accompanied by severe, crampy abdominal pains.

Children with acute infectious diarrhea are contagious and may require a short period of isolation.

What about children with chronic diarrhea?

Chronic diarrhea can also be of infectious origin. Parasites such as *Giardia* and *Dientamoeba fragilis* are common in day-care populations (affecting 10 to 15 percent of children), though many children carrying these parasites have no symptoms. Noninfectious causes of chronic diarrhea include ulcerative colitis, Crohn's disease, lactase deficiency, malabsorption, cystic fibrosis, celiac disease, disaccharidase deficiency, Hirschsprung's disease, and food allergy. Diarrhea that lasts more than three to four days with no sign of improvement should be reported to your child's doctor, even if the child seems well otherwise.

Drinking too much fruit juice is a common cause of chronic diarrhea in toddlers, and promptly ceases when the fruit juice is discontinued. The high concentration of sugar causes excess fluid to be poured into the intestine. Diluting the fruit juice half and half with water should lead to an improvement in the diarrhea if this is the cause.

How is acute diarrhea treated?

The treatment of acute diarrhea of an infectious origin in non-hospitalized children is always controversial. The goal is to correct any fluid loss, as well as any electrolyte imbalance, and at the same time provide adequate nutrition.

Antibiotics do not help acute viral diarrhea, but can be used to treat certain types of bacterial diarrhea and the diarrhea caused by certain parasites.

Diarrhea medicines that can be obtained without prescription are not advisable for children under three years of age, and should be used with a great deal of caution even with older children. These agents do not repair the injury to the intestinal wall and may actually make things worse by masking the symptoms and persuading you to feed your child before the child has recovered enough. The process causing the diarrhea may worsen, with continuing losses of salt and water, while you may feel that your child is better because you see less diarrhea.

The course of action currently recommended when your child has acute diarrhea is to give an oral electrolyte solution (see above) in the first twenty-four hours. For breast-feeding infants, breast milk may be continued. Once the diarrhea slows down (usually within twenty-four hours), the child can receive age-appropriate solid foods, followed by milk or formula in forty-eight to seventy-two hours if the improvement continues. Solids include complex carbohydrates for older children—bread, pasta, rice, potato—and applesauce, bananas, and cereals containing rice for infants. Fluid in doses of 30 mL (2 tablespoons) per half-hour is suggested; gradually increase the amount as the child tolerates more.

In the case of prolonged or severe diarrhea, milk or formula low in lactose may be necessary for a short period, until the bowel has repaired itself. Boiled skim milk should never be used to treat diarrhea (or even given to normal children). Drink mixes and soft drinks are not ideal as they are low in electrolytes. Gatorade may be used for children older than three to four years. Popsicles or anything cold (even fluids from the refrigerator) may make diarrhea worse; one study showed that the intestine moves more quickly when the stomach is exposed to cold.

Call your doctor if the diarrhea is increasing in amount despite treatment, especially if the child continues to have a fever and keeps vomiting. If the diarrhea does not improve in twenty-four to thirty-six hours after oral-electrolyte treatment, or persists after three to five days, maintain close contact with your doctor's office.

CHAPTER 8

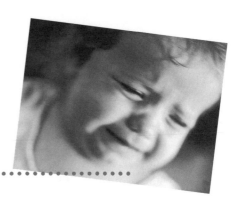

Painful Urination

• •

Pain or discomfort on urination is a frequent complaint in children and adolescents, on its own or in combination with other complaints such as genital itching or pain, fever, difficulty urinating, and frequent urination. Infants and young children who can't complain in words may show signs of pain during urination by crying, drawing up their legs, and/or clutching at their genitals. Parents may notice changes in children's genitals (such as redness or swelling); changes in the smell or color of the urine; vaginal discharge or bleeding; or abnormalities in the stream of urine, such as very frequent small urinations, or a weak, dribbling urine stream.

Fortunately, many of the minor changes parents notice are within the wide range of normal behavior and urine characteristics, and don't indicate an illness or problem. For example, a young girl who complains of mild itching or burning during one episode of urination but not during subsequent urinations is likely to be perfectly well when assessed by a physician. Similarly, parents may notice that their apparently healthy young boy is urinating more frequently and gets up once in the night to urinate after days when he's had large amounts of liquids, but not on other days. There are no simple guidelines that tell exactly when a minor change in urine habits means a real problem, but many physicians believe the following signs call for prompt medical advice:

• genital pain, swelling, discolouration, or tenderness;

• pain or burning during urination that is either persistent, or severe enough to cause crying or upset, or associated with fever;

• definite changes in the colour of urine, such as urine that appears pink, red, or "cola" in color;

- any changes in urination habits accompanied by abdominal or back pain, weight loss, appetite loss, vomiting, or lethargy.

Signs that likely call for medical advice, though not so urgently, may include:

- mild burning, itching, or discomfort during urination that doesn't occur with every urination;

- minor changes in urination habits (increased frequency, new onset of getting up to urinate at night);

- persistent wetting of clothes during the day, or bedwetting (in a child who has been previously dry), which is not accompanied by pain or other signs of illness.

What causes painful urination?

There are many causes, and the significance depends very much on the age, sex, and circumstances of the child. The presence or absence of other complaints is often very important in helping to determine the cause and importance of the painful urination. The most common causes are vulvitis in girls, urinary-tract infection in boys and girls, and balanoposthitis in boys. "Vulvitis" is irritation or infection of the sensitive, moist lining of the external female genitals, the vulva. "Balanoposthitis" refers to irritation and/or infection of the sensitive moist lining of the tip of the penis and under the foreskin. Sometimes painful urination is clearly attributable to other causes, such as a bruise from an injury, a sexually transmitted infection, or passage of a urinary stone. Only very rarely do doctors have to consider causes such as a foreign object placed in the child's urethra (the tube that drains urine from the bladder), a partial blockage of the urethra, and so on.

How serious is a urinary-tract infection?

The term "urinary-tract infection" refers to a bacterial infection of the urine and lining or organs of the urinary tract, the bladder, and/or the kidneys. The complaints associated with infected urine vary tremendously, and may be as mild and simple as burning with urination or as severe as fever, vomiting, abdominal pain, and lethargy. Since most such infections occur in children younger than three years of age, who may not be able to communicate pain on voiding, many infections are brought to the parents' attention by fever or other signs, rather than complaints of pain. It is not necessary to check the urine for infection every time a child has a fever, but infants less than six months old with fever, children with fever and abdominal pain or changes in urination, and children with fever but no obvious explanation such as a cough and runny nose should probably have their urine tested.

About urine tests

A urinary-tract infection is diagnosed when bacteria are found growing in urine obtained directly from the bladder. In older children, a sample is caught from the middle of a urine stream with a special sterile container, after the child's genitals have been gently washed and rinsed with clean water. This urine must be refrigerated immediately, and delivered to the laboratory as soon as possible. Urine caught in a non-sterile container, or in another way, such as with a urine bag stuck to the child's genital area, is likely to be contaminated, and may suggest an infection when none exists.

In younger children, where a mid-stream sample can't be obtained, a sample may have to be taken through special techniques such as introducing a very small, soft plastic tube (catheter) into the bladder through the urethra. While this may appear painful, it's often necessary in order to establish whether or not an infection exists. Since a urinary-tract infection may prompt several other actions, such as X-ray examinations—one of which may involve introducing a catheter into the bladder—it's clearly important to be certain about the diagnosis.

Children with bacterial infection of the urine can be roughly divided into three groups: those without any symptoms; those with inflammation and infection of the bladder; and those with inflammation and infection of the kidney. Young girls sometimes have bacterial growth in their urine without ever feeling unwell. In most cases this form of infection doesn't appear to cause any damage and doesn't require treatment, so there's no point doing a urine test on an apparently healthy child with no complaints of pain, fever, or urination problems. However, it's important to diagnose infections that cause these complaints and involve the bladder or kidneys. If they are left untreated or recur frequently, they may cause scarring and damage to the kidneys.

A simple abnormality called "vesicoureteral reflux" may be found in up to a third of children with urinary-tract infection. Reflux means that some urine flushes back up to the kidneys when the bladder is emptied. This makes it more difficult for the body to keep the urine free from infection, so these children often have repeated urine infections. Reflux itself doesn't damage the kidneys or cause any complaints or symptoms. The vast majority of children with reflux live their lives with normal kidney function, and it's important not to give them unnecessary anxiety or a sense that they have kidney disease. However, those who have repeated or severe urine infections may end up with kidney injury, which sometimes results in problems such as high blood pressure. Other abnormalities of the kidneys or drainage system are also found, but these are rare.

Significant kidney injury following urinary-tract infections, with or without reflux, is extremely rare in children who are otherwise well. However, infants with urinary-tract infections, children with repeated infections, or children with other problems, such as poor growth or persistent problems with urinating, are probably at greater risk. These children may benefit from X-ray tests looking for abnormalities such as vesicoureteral reflux. It is not yet clear whether all children with their first urinary-tract infection benefit from these tests.

How are urinary-tract infections treated?

Children with proven urinary-tract infections that cause symptoms such as painful urination require antibiotics. In most cases these can be given by mouth, but young infants, or children with severe infection or problems such as vomiting, will require admission to hospital for antibiotic treatment. Children whose X-ray studies show abnormalities of the kidney drainage system, or who have repeated urine infections, appear to benefit from longer-term daily antibiotic treatment. This treatment—for six months or longer, depending on the problem—helps prevent repeat infections. Some children with urinary-tract infections have problems with frequent urination and daytime wetting that persist after treatment of the infection. Though many physicians suggest bladder-training exercises for these children (see Chapter 6, "Toilet Training"), no one knows whether these exercises prevent repeated infections.

What are the signs of vulvitis?

Vulvitis (or vulvovaginitis, when the vagina is also involved) can usually be seen on examination, as the vulva becomes red and sore to touch, and sometimes has a discharge. Aside from the itching and burning that often persist between urinations, and the discharge, vulvovaginitis does not involve other difficulties such as changes in urination habits or urine, fever, or other signs of illness.

Prior to puberty the surface of the vulva is thin and more susceptible to irritation and inflammation. Young girls often have brief recurrent episodes of vulvitis, apparently because irritants and moisture are trapped in the vulva. This is called "nonspecific" vulvitis. Sensitivity to soaps and perfumes, and the use of tight clothing or diapers that trap moisture, may account for some of the irritation. Some girls seem particularly prone to vulvitis during and following toilet training; poor habits in cleaning the child's bottom may be part of the cause (see below).

Nonspecific vulvitis is a concern mainly because of the discomfort it causes. However, over a period of time, chronic inflammation may cause changes such as labial agglutination, in which the *labia minora*, the thin flaps of tissue on either side of the urethral and vaginal openings, stick together. This may cause pain with urination, and the labia may bleed if attempts are made to pull them apart, but separation can usually be achieved with treatment.

Vulvitis may also be caused by a specific infection, such as group A streptococcus, the organism that causes "strep throat," or by a yeast called "candida." Pinworms, short thread-like parasitic worms that live in the intestines, may occasionally infect a young child and cause anal itching, burning, and/or vulvitis.

Once adolescent girls reach puberty, they appear less susceptible to irritants and moisture trapping, and are more likely to get the kinds of vulvovaginitis that occur in adult women. Perfumed sanitary pads, tampons, and other feminine-hygiene products may act as irritants for girls this age.

How is vulvitis prevented and treated?

No particular routine has been tested or proven to work, but the following general steps are unlikely to cause harm, and experience suggests that they may prevent nonspecific vulvitis, or promote healing.

- Use bath products carefully. Avoid bubble baths and perfumed bath or hygiene products, excessive use of shampoo or soap in the bathwater, and applying soap directly to the membranes of the vulva.

- Use frequent baths in plain, tepid water, followed by gentle drying, and give the vulval area a chance to air-dry after the bath. While the child still has discomfort, she may feel better having several baths a day, and may even be encouraged to urinate while sitting in the bath if urination causes significant pain.

- Select loose day and night clothing to promote circulation of air and to prevent restriction and trapping of moisture and irritants.

- Carefully supervise toileting hygiene. Avoid contaminating the vulva with soiled toilet paper; always wipe from front to back, *away* from the vulva.

When vulvitis is severe, doesn't respond to simple measures, or is associated with a large amount of discharge (suggesting vulvovaginitis), the physician will look for specific causes. The urine may be tested to ensure that no urinary-tract infection is present, and the child will be examined and perhaps given a few simple tests. If there are signs of vulvitis from germs such as group A streptococcus, candida, or pinworms, she will clearly benefit from antibiotics. However, if the bacteria found on the surface of the vulva are normally present in girls without vulvitis, antibiotics are unlikely to do any good. If your child has severe or long-lasting vulvitis and labial agglutination, an estrogen cream can be prescribed to assist in healing and separating the labia.

Girls with symptoms of vulvitis or vulvovaginitis who have engaged in sexual activity, or who may have been victims of sexual assault, require special assessment by a physician familiar with these problems. In this case, pain with urination or vulvitis requires a diligent approach that includes a search for sexually transmitted infections such as chlamydia and gonorrhea, as well as counseling for prevention of pregnancy and sexually transmitted diseases (including AIDS and hepatitis).

What about the problems boys have?

Uncircumcised boys occasionally develop inflammation of the membranes of the foreskin and the tip of the penis (the glans) covered by the foreskin. This is called "balanoposthitis," and it usually causes pain and swelling of the tip of the penis, in addition to painful urination. In some cases this condition appears without any obvious cause. If there is white or gray discharge from under the foreskin, the inflammation is due to infection. Sometimes attempts to force back a foreskin that doesn't retract easily irritate the membranes and cause painful urination—or a painful swollen glans and difficult or painful urination can be caused when a foreskin with a relatively tight opening is pulled back and becomes trapped around the base of the glans. Once the glans begins to swell, this condition, called "paraphimosis," can rapidly become extremely painful; it requires medical advice as soon as possible.

Balanoposthitis is effectively treated with antibiotics by mouth. Paraphimosis requires a physician to perform a special manoeuvre to get the foreskin back over the glans, perhaps with sedation or pain medication. For all these conditions, hygiene and comfort are best achieved by frequent, tepid, plain-water baths, and urination should be encouraged with the child sitting in the bath if urination is still painful.

Boys who have been circumcised may also have problems with painful urination. Occasionally they develop irritation and bleeding around the tip of the penis, at the opening of the urethra, called "meatal ulceration." This generally occurs in young boys who are still in diapers, or in boys who frequently wet their clothing. The irritation appears to be caused by contact with urine trapped in the diaper or clothing. Treatment with skin protectants such as petrolatum, and attention to maintaining hygiene and minimizing moisture and urine exposure, may reduce the problem.

Q Does circumcision avoid problems, or cause them?

Some medical problems, such as urinary-tract infections and adult cancer of the penis, may occur more frequently in uncircumcised males. In addition to this, problems such as balanoposthitis and paraphimosis occur only in uncircumcised boys. Also, circumcised adult males are thought to have less risk of developing sexually transmitted diseases, including AIDS. Because of these concerns some physicians recommend circumcision of boys at birth. However, it's not at all clear whether circumcision can be justified for health reasons. For example, cancer of the penis is an extraordinarily rare condition that occurs much later in adulthood. Urinary-tract infections may be more prevalent in uncircumcised boys, but they are still uncommon and easy to treat, and there is no proof at all that they put uncircumcised boys at any higher risk of kidney scarring or other health problems. Even though circumcision is a relatively simple procedure, with few complications, the pain and risk of those complications (excessive bleeding, infection, and poor healing with scarring) must be balanced against the limited potential benefit.

However, certain boys may benefit from circumcision or related surgery. Those who have had an episode of balanoposthitis or paraphimosis may get it again, and may therefore benefit from circumcision. As well, a very small number of boys may benefit because the foreskin opening is so tight (called "phimosis") that urination is messy or difficult, or retraction can't be achieved in adolescence. The decision must take many factors into account: how constant the problem is, the number of times it has occurred, the severity of the problem, and so on.

Some parents have social or religious reasons for circumcising their boys. Complications from the procedure are rare enough, and mostly mild enough, that such reasons are usually considered an acceptable basis for circumcision. Still, the procedure is not trivial, and not without some pain, even for newborn infants. There is evidence that medications such as local anesthetics can significantly reduce the pain, and many doctors regard these as a necessary component of good medical care.

The issue of female circumcision

There is currently no proof that circumcision does any significant long-lasting harm, psychologically or physically, to most males. Female circumcision, which involves cutting away parts of the vulva and often includes sewing the opening of the vagina closed, or nearly closed, is a totally different procedure. Female circumcision can cause significant complications and suffering, both following the circumcision and throughout life. Because of this—despite the fact that female circumcision is culturally important in some societies—many medical organizations have taken a strong stand against the procedure, considering it unethical, and a case of malpractice for a physician to participate in performing it.

 Does circumcision make hygiene easier?

Bathing and hygiene of boys, circumcised or not, is not necessarily complicated. Though the connection is not as common or as obvious as with girls, nonspecific irritants such as soaps and the trapping of moisture, or poor hygiene with toileting, may contribute to irritation of the glans. The same general approaches used with girls, such as loose clothing with adequate air circulation to ensure drying, may be of use with boys. At birth the foreskin cannot easily be pulled back over the glans. However, as boys age the foreskin gradually becomes more mobile, and by three years of age it can usually be pulled back. However, regularly pulling the foreskin back or cleaning under it while bathing the child serves no clear purpose for most boys and may occasionally cause additional irritation and problems.

Sexually transmitted infections can occur in sexually active or abused boys. Boys with painful urination who have been sexually active require assessment by a physician able to deal with the multiple issues involved. Finally, testicular pain and/or swelling may occasionally be experienced by boys, though these conditions rarely involve painful urination. Unless these are brief, mild conditions obviously caused by minor injury, they require prompt medical advice.

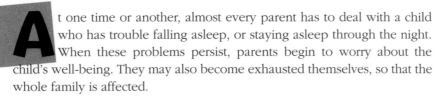

CHAPTER 9

Sleeping Patterns and Problems

At one time or another, almost every parent has to deal with a child who has trouble falling asleep, or staying asleep through the night. When these problems persist, parents begin to worry about the child's well-being. They may also become exhausted themselves, so that the whole family is affected.

We still don't know exactly why we need to sleep, but we do know that people deprived of sleep become cranky and don't think very clearly.

We divide sleep into two main types—REM (rapid eye movement) sleep, during which we dream, and non-REM sleep, which makes us rested. Non-REM sleep varies from very light to very deep. During the night we go through repeated cycles of sleep, from light non-REM into deeper and deeper non-REM, and then into REM sleep and dreams. Between these cycles, we sometimes have brief periods of being awake.

A baby's cycle through the stages of non-REM sleep and then REM sleep and possible awakening generally takes fifty to sixty minutes. By adulthood this cycle lengthens to some ninety minutes. Babies spend about half their sleep time dreaming, but this declines as they get older; adolescents—like adults—dream for about 20 percent of their sleep time.

Children differ widely in the amount of sleep they need. The average baby sleeps about sixteen hours out of twenty-four, a one-year-old about fourteen hours, a three-year-old about twelve hours. Under six months of age most children have three or four daytime naps a day, from six to twelve months they have about two naps, and sometime between three and four years of age they drop the daytime nap completely.

If you are hoping to change your child's sleep pattern, begin keeping a sleep diary to record the present pattern and any changes that develop. This way, you'll know if you're making progress. You'll find a sample sleep diary at the end of this chapter.

Q Why is it so hard to get some children to go to sleep?

If you have a toddler, you've probably faced endless bedtime requests for a drink of water, a trip to the bathroom, and so on. Difficulty in getting a child settled at night is a very common problem. Fortunately, it can usually be resolved with a structured bedtime routine.

The routine should last fifteen to twenty minutes and should be the same every night. For example, the child goes to the bathroom, completes tooth-brushing and face-washing, and gets into bed for a bedtime story; at the end of the story you turn out the light, give the child a good-night hug and kiss, and leave. A structured routine like this is very reassuring to a child and means that both you and the child know what is expected and allowed.

Q But what if my child won't go to sleep in bed alone?

Once your child develops the habit of falling asleep under certain circum-stances—such as in your arms, or in front of the television—you'll have to work to gradually modify that pattern and create the structured routine you want (see the discussion of maladaptive sleep associations, below).

Q What about a child who keeps waking up during the night?

Several studies have shown that it's common for children to wake up at night, especially between the ages of one and four; 10 percent of this age group awaken at least twice a night, and 30 percent at least three times a week. But the problem is not the fact that the child awakens—awakening between sleep cycles is normal, as noted earlier—but that he or she doesn't go back to sleep. These "night awakenings" are the most common sleep dis-order in children.

Unfortunately, night awakenings can be very persistent, and they often don't go away on their own; one study showed that four out of ten children who had a problem with night awakenings at age eight months still had it at three years. The awakenings have been associated with several factors: dif-ficulties at birth, developmental problems, parental depression, family stress, and the child having a difficult temperament.

Your response to a night awakening can also be an important factor. If you "reward" the child—with a feeding, for example, or by bringing him or her back to your own bed, or by any other soothing contact—you're sending the child a message that waking up at night brings comfort and companionship. This is positive reinforcement of the waking-up habit.

Another factor in night awakenings is sleep associations—the bedtime conditions that the child typically falls asleep with. If these are conditions that he or she can't recreate alone, the normal awakenings that can come several times a night become traps that the child can't escape. Examples of such "maladaptive" sleep associations include:

- being rocked in your arms;

- breast-feeding or bottle-feeding;

- being in another room or someone else's bed;

- using a pacifier the child can't replace;

- listening to music the child can't restart.

Often, positive reinforcement and maladaptive sleep associations combine to keep a child waking up. For example, a little boy falls asleep with a pacifier that rolls out of reach. When he has a normal nighttime awakening, he can't get back to sleep without the pacifier; he starts to fuss, and in comes a parent to retrieve the pacifier and soothe him with back rubs and a lullaby. Is it any wonder he keeps waking up?

Preventing night awakenings

The key to preventing night awakenings is teaching your child to fall asleep alone at an early age. Even a baby ten or twelve weeks old can be put into a crib or cradle awake. To avoid creating positive reinforcement for waking,

- keep nighttime encounters short and boring

- don't do unnecessary diaper changes at night

- try to drop nighttime feedings after six months of age

- follow a consistent bedtime routine at the same time every evening

Q What can I do if my child already has poor sleep habits?

Several studies have shown that behavior management is quite effective in treating frequent night awakenings. The basic principles are:

1. identify the maladaptive sleep associations, and teach the child to fall asleep alone in circumstances he or she can re-create later in the night;

2. identify and gradually remove any positive reinforcement ("reward") for night awakenings.

In one study, parents of four-month-olds were encouraged to start putting their babies to bed partially awake so that they could learn to fall asleep by themselves; at nine months of age the babies were sleeping significantly better than a control group whose parents had not received such advice. In another study, the principles of teaching the child to sleep alone and removing positive reinforcers were applied to nineteen children under the age of five who had a history of frequent night awakenings; researchers reported an 84 percent success rate, which was still maintained six months after the study ended.

 Does that mean I should just leave the baby crying?

Letting a child "cry it out" makes sense in terms of behavior modification, as it removes the positive reinforcement of parental soothing and also leaves the child to get back to sleep without any maladaptive associations (food, pacifier, etc.). One study divided children with night awakenings into two groups; the parents of Group 1 were told to leave their children crying, and the parents of Group 2 were simply put on a waiting list for treatment. The number of night awakenings in Group 1 decreased by 50 percent in the first week, and by 75 percent in the second week. However, some of the parents withdrew from the study when they learned that this was one of the treatments. In short, letting your baby "cry it out" often works, but not all parents can bear to do it.

 Are there more gradual ways to change my child's behavior?

You can take things one at a time. Start by writing down your own analysis of the sleep problem: both the maladaptive sleep associations and the positive reinforcers. (For an example, see the sidebar "Changing Johnny's sleep habits.") This will give you a clear idea of what you need to change. Then tackle one new item every week or two.

It's essential that parents work together on this; it's difficult to deal with a screaming child *and* a screaming adult in the middle of the night!

Changing Johnny's sleep habits

Johnny is fourteen months old. At nine months he started waking regularly at night, and now he's up three times a night. He goes to sleep well at bedtime; his parents hold him in a rocker and give him a bottle and move him to his crib once he's asleep. When he wakes up at night, they find that if they give him a bottle of formula he'll go back to sleep in five or ten minutes; he generally finishes two eight-ounce bottles a night. Because they're exhausted by this regimen, his parents have recently started bringing him into bed with them.

Analysis of sleep problem

Maladaptive associations

- falling asleep on bottle
- falling asleep outside crib

Positive reinforcers

- nighttime feeding
- moving to parents' bed

Once Johnny's parents have analyzed the problem, they can start changing their son's habits. First they gradually decrease his nighttime feedings; then, step by step, they move him towards falling asleep in his own bed with no bottle, and staying there.

 How do I go about cutting out nighttime feedings?

Healthy children over the age of six months don't need food at night. If this is one of the things you have to change, do it first; it's hard to make other behavioral changes when your child is looking for food. Make changes gradually, over one or two weeks.

If your child is on bottles, decrease the contents of each bottle by one ounce each night; for example, two eight-ounce bottles on Monday, two seven-ounce bottles Tuesday, and so on, until you reach zero. This method is easier than watering down the formula, which leaves you with a child expecting water every night.

If your child is breast-fed, decrease the feeding time by one or two minutes a night; you can also lengthen the time between feeds by half an hour per night. Again, don't try to change other sleep habits until you've finished changing the feeding habits.

How do I get my child to fall asleep alone, if I can't bear to ignore the crying?

You can retrain your child by simply waiting a little longer each day before going in. This works best in a child under two who is still sleeping in a crib. (Don't use this method if your child is old enough to fall out of the crib.) Go through your normal bedtime routine and then put the child in the crib awake. Leave the room, but come back from time to time to reassure the child until he or she falls asleep—but stay only a minute or two each time, and don't pick the child up. Wait a little longer after each visit, and increase the intervals from night to night. For example:

	1st wait	*2nd wait*	*3rd wait*	*further waits*
Day 1	2 min.	4 min.	6 min.	6 min.
Day 2	4 min.	6 min.	8 min.	8 min.
Day 3	6 min.	8 min.	10 min.	10 min.
Day 4	8 min.	10 min.	12 min.	12 min.

Most children are quite upset during the first few nights of this change, but soon learn to fall asleep alone. The same technique can be used to decrease your response when the child wakes up during the night.

But what if my child is already sleeping in a bed?

If you try the above method with an older child, he or she may follow you when you leave the room. Instead, you can try "chair sitting." Begin by sitting in a chair close to the child's bed—don't talk, just be there—and move the chair a foot farther away each night, until you're out of the room and down the hall. Children are rarely upset by this, as the change is so gradual. If a child does get up and follow you, give a warning the first time; after that, you can go out and hold the door closed for one minute and then return. If the child continues to follow you, increase the time you hold the door shut, until he or she stays quietly in bed.

Before you start this routine, explain the plan to the child; you may want to mark the final destination of your chair on the floor with masking tape. If the child is over three years old, it may help to offer a sticker as a reward for each night of cooperation.

If I cut out daytime naps, is my child more likely to sleep through the night?

Daytime naps generally shouldn't be more than two or three hours. Review your sleep diary. If your child is napping too much, gradually reducing nap time by five or ten minutes a day may increase nighttime sleeping. As a rule, children should be up by 8:00 A.M., and afternoon naps for those over a year old should end by 4:00 P.M.

Can I give my child sleeping medications?

Sleeping medications should not generally be used for children with night awakenings. They're effective, but once you take the child off the medication the problem usually starts again. Changing the child's behavior patterns provides a lasting "cure" and doesn't have the potential side effects of medication.

What do I do if my child has nightmares?

Children sleep lightly during REM (dream) sleep, and may wake up screaming from nightmares. Bad dreams are especially distressing to toddlers, who can't understand the difference between dreams and reality. A child who is old enough to talk may be able to describe parts of the dream to you, so you can discuss it. In any case, your presence and reassurance will be comforting.

Recurrent nightmares are usually a sign that something is bothering the child; it may be minor, or something significant. With an older child, you can try talking about likely issues during the daytime, to relieve the stress. If the problem seems serious, consult your doctor.

What if the child is screaming in terror but doesn't seem awake?

Imagine that your child has been asleep for a couple of hours when you hear a blood-curdling scream. You rush to the nursery and find the child sitting up, dripping with sweat, heart pounding. If the eyes are open, they look glazed and the pupils are dilated. Yet when you talk to the child you get no response. This is not a nightmare; it's a night terror.

Night terrors—which are classified as "disorders of arousal"—happen when a child is in *non-dream* sleep, moving from a deeper stage to a lighter stage. No one really knows what causes them, but they're common in children aged three to six and gradually decrease after that. Though the child may be sitting up and wide-eyed, he or she is *not awake*, and is not aware of the surroundings. The episode may last as long as twenty or thirty minutes before the child falls back into "peaceful" sleep. He or she will have no recollection of the terror the next morning.

Night terrors tend to come in clumps; there may be one or two a week for three or four months, and then they may disappear. There may be another series sometime later. A study of children who had recurring night terrors before the age of ten found that, on average, they continued for 3.9 years. It also found that the children were emotionally normal. Night terrors tend to run in families.

What can I do about a night terror?

The first rule is to remain calm. Night terrors are very upsetting for parents, but remember: the child is asleep and will not remember this in the morning. Satisfy yourself that this is in fact a night terror; if the child is awake, the event was probably a nightmare. Night terrors can be confused with nighttime seizures, but children with seizures also have them in the daytime, and seizures often include urinating.

If it's a true night terror, stay in the room until it's over, and move breakables out of the way, but don't try to waken the child as this may prolong the episode. No further treatment is usually necessary, but if the episodes seem atypical, or a cycle lasts more than four months, you may want to consult your doctor.

Why do some children walk and talk in their sleep?

Like night terrors, sleepwalking and sleeptalking are disorders of arousal, and occur as the child moves from deep non-REM sleep to a lighter stage. The child usually wanders aimlessly and talks incoherently, and doesn't remember the episode the next day.

Because the child is asleep, he or she is unaware of danger, so it's up to you to take precautions. Supervise the child until he or she goes back to sleep, but don't try to wake the child up, as this may cause agitation. If you know a child sleepwalks, be sure doors and windows are securely locked, and take measures against any other hazards.

Most sleepwalkers are ten to twelve years of age; sometimes sleepwalking begins as night terrors come to an end. There's usually a history of sleepwalking in the family. The condition doesn't seem to be linked to any emotional disorders, and no medical treatment is required.

Why do some babies rock and bang their heads when they're sleepy?

Rocking and head-banging are very common in young children, particularly boys; the behavior tends to start after six months of age and disappears a few months later, but it sometimes goes on until the child is four or five.

Children usually rock by swinging back and forth in a crawling position. Those who bang their heads may also be in that position, or may be sitting up. Both behaviors are most common at bedtime, when the child is drowsy, but may also occur during the day or during a night awakening.

We don't know why some children bang their heads, but the actions may reflect the fact that rhythmic movements are soothing. The banging doesn't injure the child, although it may be hard on the walls and furniture. Almost all young head-bangers are emotionally well and developing normally. Although head-banging is more frequent in children with neurological problems such as autism and mental retardation, such conditions are usually obvious from daytime behavior. There have been isolated cases of older head-bangers with emotional difficulties, but no good studies have been done.

There are no reported studies on treatment of head-banging. Most pediatricians recommend ignoring the behavior, since it does no harm and eventually goes away; in any case, it's very hard to stop the child from doing it. If your child continues head-banging past the age of five, you should see your doctor, who can review the child's health and emotional status and look for any stresses or anxieties.

When to see your doctor about sleep disorders

Sleep disorders are common in children, and most go away without treatment, but a few situations call for medical advice:

- persistent snoring or mouth-breathing
- night terrors lasting over four months
- persistent nightmares
- head-banging past five years of age
- concern about the child's emotional or general development

Sleep Diary

Please keep a record of your child's sleep patterns both day and night.

✗ – child put to bed

✓ – asleep

	Night		A.M.		Morning		P.M.	
	8 9 10 11 12	1 2 3 4 5	6 7 8 9 10 11 12	1 2 3 4 5 6 7				
Week # ____				
Sunday				
Monday				
Tuesday				
Wednesday				
Thursday				
Friday				
Saturday				
Week # ____				
Sunday				
Monday				
Tuesday				
Wednesday				
Thursday				
Friday				
Saturday				
Week # ____				
Sunday				
Monday				
Tuesday				
Wednesday				
Thursday				
Friday				
Saturday				

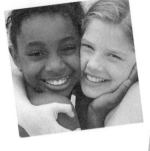
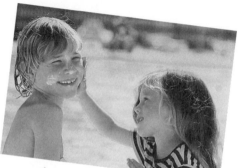

CHAPTER 10

Skin: Spots and Rashes

•••

kin problems are relatively common in children, and are often the cause of much parental concern. However, the vast majority are not serious. Many rashes don't bother the infant or child in the least, and most will disappear with no treatment. But some rashes are associated with serious diseases, and call for medical attention.

Q **What spots and rashes do newborns get?**

Chapter 2 described milia (like white or yellow pimples) and erythema toxicum (like red-rimmed pimples), which normally disappear soon after birth.

Mongolian spots are dark, pigmented patches of skin, usually on the lower back, buttocks, and legs. They are very common in Indian, Asian, and black children but may occur in any race. They tend to fade with age. No complications are associated with them, and no treatment is necessary.

Vasomotor instability is often found in newborns and young infants. In this condition, the baby's skin may turn deep purple or red during crying; the hands and feet frequently look bluish, and the skin may be mottled. If the infant is otherwise well and vigorous, this is not a cause for concern.

Hemangiomas are abnormal collections of blood vessels that take several forms. The most common are "salmon patches," flat, pale pink "birthmarks" on the back of the neck (sometimes called "stork bites"), eyelids, forehead ("angel's kiss"), and nose. Those on the face usually fade and disappear by age two or three; those on the neck may not, but since they are usually covered by hair they are not unsightly.

"Port-wine stains" are flat, pink or reddish purple lesions, usually on the face. Since they don't fade, they may be a significant cosmetic problem. Laser therapy has recently been shown to be a safe and effective treatment for many port-wine stains.

"Strawberry" (capillary) hemangiomas are not usually present at birth, but appear within the first few weeks of life and may grow for several months. They are raised red or purplish marks that can occur anywhere on the face, body, or limbs. More than 90 percent will shrink and disappear partially or completely without leaving scars, so treatment is usually not indicated, but patience is very important. Medical intervention is sometimes necessary—if, for example, the hemangioma interferes with vision or breathing. Very rarely, these hemangiomas bleed or become infected.

 ### What other skin problems do small babies get?

Seborrheic dermatitis looks like yellow greasy scales, sometimes crusted. When it occurs on the scalp, it's known as "cradle cap." This rash may also occur in the creases of the diaper area and neck, and under the arms, and occasionally it affects the face. In these areas the rash often has a red, inflamed appearance, but it's not itchy or painful. Seborrheic dermatitis usually starts around four weeks of age, and has usually cleared up by one year.

Treatment is with moisturizing creams or ointments. If the "cradle cap" is very bad and shows no improvement, tar or salicylic acid–based shampoos may occasionally be applied (these should be used sparingly and carefully in infants). Keep in mind that seborrheic dermatitis bothers you much more than it bothers your baby! Other skin areas usually respond to steroid creams, which should be applied under the direction of a physician.

A word about steroids

Steroids are cortisone-like medications that are often prescribed for skin problems. They are quite different from the steroids (androgens) that are used illegally by people trying to improve their strength or sporting abilities. Steroids used for medical purposes are available as skin creams, and as tablets or liquids to be taken by mouth. (Intravenous and inhaled steroids are also available, but these are seldom used for skin problems.) When prescribed and used appropriately, steroids are both safe and effective.

Diaper rashes include several different rashes that occur in the area covered by diapers. The rashes most frequently seen are "diaper dermatitis" and "candida dermatitis."

"Diaper dermatitis" is probably due to pressure and irritation in the diaper region. It starts as shiny, reddish spots that may spread, join together, and become raw and painful. The skin creases are not usually involved. Diaper dermatitis usually appears in infants age three to twelve months, and prevention is easier than cure. The following measures may be helpful:

- Change diapers as frequently as possible (and reasonable), especially if the baby already has a rash or diarrhea, or if you are using cloth diapers.

- Avoid tight-fitting diapers.

- Avoid irritating soaps; wash the skin with warm water only.

- Try to keep the skin dry.

Barrier creams containing zinc oxide are most useful after a rash has set in. Once the baby is out of diapers, this rash will not recur.

"Candida dermatitis" (thrush) is due to a yeast, which thrives in warm moist environments such as the diaper area. It can also occur in other areas, including the mouth. In the diaper area, it starts in the creases and spreads outward. Little pimples or pustules are often seen at the edges; the rash itself is often red and raw. Some babies develop candida diaper rashes after taking oral antibiotics.

Treatment is with antifungal creams. Some doctors recommend using a steroid cream in combination with an antifungal agent, but no studies have been done to determine which is the best method of treatment. Oral medications are not necessary unless there is evidence of thrush in the baby's mouth.

Babies with frequently recurring candida infections, or infections that don't clear up with treatment, should be seen by a physician.

 Why do some babies have patches of different skin color?
Normal skin color is mainly due to a pigment called "melanin." Uneven skin color can result from too much or too little pigment in small or large areas of the body. These may be present at birth or develop later. In some people, injuries heal with areas of increased or decreased pigment. Aside from the cosmetic aspect, most abnormalities of pigment are not a cause for concern. Sometimes, though, they are associated with underlying illnesses, or increased risk of certain diseases. For this reason, it's a good idea to point out areas of different skin color to your doctor.

Why do some babies have a lot of body hair?

The vast majority of children who appear "hairy" are quite normal. Frequently, other members of their family are hairy too. There is a large variation in the amount of body hair between different racial and ethnic groups. Western society, unfortunately, favors less body hair, particularly in women—hence the large market for hair-removing products.

Occasionally, diseases cause excess body hair. In some cases the illness is obvious (for example, severe malnutrition or anorexia nervosa can result in increased hairiness). As well, some medications cause increased body hair. If the increased hair growth is all over the body, it is called "hypertrichosis." If it's in the genital area, under the arms, or on the face, it is called "hirsutism."

You should be concerned about your child having too much body hair only if there is any indication the child may be ill, or if hirsutism occurs in a child who is too young to be entering puberty.

Aren't some rashes caused by allergies?

Atopic dermatitis (eczema) is by definition an extremely itchy skin rash. It can occur in all age groups, but is more common in infants and young children and usually starts within the first year of life. The site and appearance of the rash vary with age: in infants the face is most often involved; in older children the crooks of the elbows and backs of the knees are typically affected. In young children the rash often looks moist, whereas in older ones the skin appears hard and thickened. Scratching may cause the rash to become infected. Itching is often provoked by changes in temperature, fabrics like wool, and some soaps. Although the cause of atopic dermatitis is unknown, it is frequently associated with asthma and allergies.

Atopic dermatitis tends to improve with age, although in about 25 percent of those affected it persists into adulthood. The most important part of treatment is preventing itching. Try to keep the child in cotton clothes, and apply moisturizing creams to the child's body after bathing. Corticosteroids are the mainstay of treatment—lotions, creams, ointments, and gels are available in varying strengths—but these should be used for as short a time as possible, as long-term use may damage the skin or have other side effects. Antihistamines may be used, especially at night; they don't appear to have a direct effect on the skin disease but do improve sleep. The newer, non-sedating antihistamines are *not* useful. To reduce scratching, keep the child's nails short. Some parents find it helpful to put mittens on the hands of small children at night. There is no scientific evidence to prove that dietary changes make any difference in the long-term outcome of atopic dermatitis, and it's difficult to tell whether short-term improvements are due to the changes in food or just to fluctuations in the disease itself. Severely restrictive diets are generally *not* recommended as they may result in malnutrition. Any adjustments to diet should be supervised by a physician.

Contact dermatitis is an allergic skin reaction to a particular substance. Common causes include poison ivy, nickel (in jewelry, zippers, or fasteners), and cosmetics. The rash usually appears at a site that has been directly exposed, although similar rashes sometimes develop in unexposed areas of skin. The affected skin is red and swollen, and blisters may form. It's extremely itchy. Allergic contact dermatitis is unusual in children under the age of five.

Treatment is by avoiding the allergen, or removing it and thoroughly washing the affected area. Cool compresses and steroid creams may be used to relieve the symptoms. In severe cases (such as a bad case of poison ivy), a doctor can prescribe further treatment.

Urticaria (hives) is another allergic response that may be due to a number of causes, including food, drugs, insect bites, and viral infections. In contrast to contact dermatitis, direct skin contact is not necessary to produce this rash; for example, some people get hives after taking an antibiotic like penicillin by mouth. The rash consists of raised pink spots with pale centers (weals), which may be quite small or very large. The rash may come and go, and the size, shape, and site of the lesions can change very rapidly. It's very itchy, and usually lasts for two or three days.

In some children the cause of hives is obvious, but in many cases the allergic agent is never found. Many children develop hives only once. Antihistamines such as Benadryl are effective treatment for hives, but if the cause is known, avoiding it obviously makes more sense.

Occasionally, hives form part of a potentially life-threatening allergic reaction. If the child appears sick or has any difficulty breathing, or has swelling of the lips or tongue, medical help should be sought urgently. You should also consult a physician if the reaction appears to be due to a medication, or if there are accompanying symptoms such as joint swelling and fever.

 What else causes an itchy red rash?

Scabies is another cause. The rash is extremely itchy, especially at night, and looks like small, reddish, raised bumps. It's caused by tiny mites (bugs) that burrow into the skin. In older children, scabies most commonly occurs between the fingers, on the inner surface of the wrists, and in the armpits, abdomen, groin, and buttocks. In children younger than two, the rash may look like little blisters, and is likely to occur on the head and neck, palms, and soles. The infection is transmitted from person to person by close contact.

The treatment of choice is permethrin cream, which appears to be the safest drug available for the purpose. The cream should be applied to the entire body below the head for children older than two years; the entire head and neck should be included for younger children. The cream should be washed off by bathing after eight to fourteen hours. It's important to follow the instructions closely. It is recommended that *all* household members be treated at the same time, and all bedding and clothing should be washed and dried at hot temperatures, to kill any remaining mites.

 ### What if my child has a rash and a fever?

Rash and fever are prominent features of many childhood infections. The vast majority are caused by viruses. It's often possible to distinguish these illnesses by differences in the rashes, and associated features such as joint pain and conjunctivitis (red, irritated eyes, with or without mucus). However, it's sometimes difficult to make a specific diagnosis, because many viruses produce similar types of diseases. The descriptions below will give you an idea of what disease your child may have; for information on the seriousness, side-effects, and treatment of these diseases, see Chapter 14, "Diseases and Medical Conditions."

A low fever soon accompanied by a rash of *raised red bumps that become little fluid-filled blisters* suggests chicken pox. The rash usually starts on the trunk and face, and then spreads to the rest of the body.

A fine pink or red rash that begins on the face and feels like sandpaper, accompanied by fever, headache, vomiting, and sore throat, likely indicates scarlet fever. A few days later, the tongue becomes red and swollen.

Fine, pale pink spots on the face and hairline, which later spread to the rest of the body and may join up into solid pink patches, suggest rubella (German measles). There may or may not be fever.

A reddish rash that spreads down from the scalp, hairline, and neck, preceded by high fever, runny nose, cough, and red eyes, probably means the child has measles. A few days later, small white spots appear in the mouth.

A bright red rash on the face, mainly the cheeks, preceded by low fever and a sore throat, suggests fifth disease. A lacy rash may appear on the limbs and trunk.

A fine pink or reddish rash that spreads from the trunk to the neck and limbs, preceded by a high fever, may mean roseola; the disease is rare in children over the age of four.

How can I tell if a rash is serious?

It's important to look at the "company a rash keeps." If a child is well, happy, and active, you needn't worry unduly about a spot or rash that he or she hasn't even noticed! There are times, however, when you should be concerned about a rash.

Seek medical help immediately if a child also has any of the following:

- a change in level of consciousness

- extreme irritability or sleepiness

- swelling of the lips or tongue

- difficulty breathing

- bleeding or bruising

- severe headache or neck pain

Seek medical help soon if a child also has any of the following:

- sores on the lips or in the mouth, eyes, or genital area

- blistering or peeling of the skin

- joint pain and/or swelling

- blood in the urine

- fever that doesn't go away within a couple of days

- pain

- ongoing vomiting and/or diarrhea

- a known immune disorder

Seek medical help before too long if any of the following occurs:

- a skin rash doesn't go away, or keeps coming back

- a mole or spot gets bigger, changes color, or bleeds

- a child has areas of increased or decreased pigmentation

- the child is not growing well

- you are concerned about the cosmetic appearance of a spot or rash

---

Q What can I do if my child has a sunburn?

The severity of sunburn ranges from mild redness of the skin, to redness with pain and swelling and sometimes blistering. If a large area of skin has been burned, the child may feel ill and have a headache, nausea, fever, and chills. The effects are usually seen six to twelve hours after overexposure to the sun, and may get worse over the next few days. Peeling of the skin frequently follows.

Treatment is aimed at keeping the child as comfortable as possible until the skin heals. Cool baths or wet compresses may be helpful. Non-prescription (0.5 percent) steroid creams may decrease the redness and swelling. Anti-inflammatory drugs such as ASA and ibuprofen may be useful, but you should discuss them with your doctor (see the note on ASA in Chapter 5). Acetaminophen can be given to provide some pain relief.

Prevention is really the key. In addition to causing painful burns, sunburn can contribute to several types of skin cancer later in life. Children under the age of six months should be kept out of the sun as much as possible; sunscreens are not recommended for this age group. For older children, current recommendations say that sunscreens with a sun protection factor (SPF) of over 15 should be applied to exposed areas thirty to sixty minutes before they go into the sun, and that the sunscreens should be reapplied every sixty to ninety minutes. After swimming or extensive perspiration, even "waterproof" sunscreens should be reapplied.

 What about unusually dry skin?

Skin dryness is due to loss of water from the outer layers of the skin. Some families have a tendency to dry skin and chapping. Environmental factors including heat, humidity, and soap also play an important role.

The areas most affected are usually the hands, arms, and shins, which may look as if they're covered by fine, flaky scales. Dry skin isn't usually irritating, although it sometimes itches. If the problem is severe, the skin may actually crack, creating painful sores.

As with sunburn, prevention is easier than cure. You can keep room temperatures as low as comfortably possible, since heat has a drying effect, and you may find humidifiers useful. (Remember to clean your humidifier regularly, as it can be a source of mold.) Children with dry skin should not be bathed more than once every two days. Try to avoid excessive exposure to soaps. (There is no scientific evidence that one soap is better than another, for normal children.) Bath oils can be added to the water, but remember that they make the bathtub slippery and dangerous. Moisturizing lotions or creams should be applied to the child's skin after bathing, while the skin is still moist.

If dry skin doesn't improve after a few weeks of the above measures, contact your doctor. Some authorities recommend moving to a subtropical climate, especially during the winter. Unfortunately, this isn't a practical option for most of us!

Is there any remedy for acne?

Acne is probably the most common skin disorder, occurring in more than 85 percent of teenagers. Although girls are affected at a younger age than boys, severe acne is more common in boys. The cause of acne is not well understood, but it's probably due to a combination of hormonal changes and infection. Acne also occurs in young babies, probably due to the mothers' hormones. There is no evidence to support the popular belief that acne is caused by certain foods (such as chocolate) or by dirt.

Several types of spots occur in acne, including blackheads, whiteheads, pimples, and cysts. Acne can be itchy or painful, and a severe case may result in scarring. The face is most commonly affected; the back, neck, chest, and shoulders may also be involved.

Treatment of acne depends on its severity and on how concerned the patient is. Some people find that exposure to the sun improves their acne; humidity and greasy ointments may be aggravating. Certain medications (most commonly hormones) can cause or worsen acne.

Benzoyl peroxide and antibiotic creams have been shown to be useful in treating acne. Exfoliating agents like tretinoin and salicylic acid, which cause irritation of the skin followed by peeling, are also used. For more severe forms of acne, adding oral antibiotics may be helpful. Isotretinoin (Accutane) is effective for very severe acne, but it can cause major birth defects if taken during pregnancy; therefore teens should be warned *never* to share their medication.

Babies with acne don't require any treatment, since the spots will disappear on their own. Acne in teenagers usually improves by the late teens or early twenties.

CHAPTER 11

Problems with Eyes and Ears

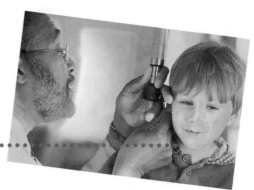

○○○○○○○○○○○○○○○○○○○○○○○○○○○○○○○○○○○○○○

Children's eyes and ears deserve special attention, not only because they are delicate and easily damaged, but also because the input they provide is essential to a child's development. Since babies can't tell us if they are seeing or hearing poorly, it's up to parents to watch for signs that their children aren't responding normally to sights and sounds.

Eye Problems

A child's eye problems sometimes begin at birth, when an eye infection may be picked up during passage through the birth canal. The eye drops given immediately after birth to prevent these infections are generally effective, but they're not infallible. Such infections can be very serious, although they respond well to treatment. If your baby has a yellowish discharge from the eyes, notify your physician.

Sometimes the eye drops themselves cause chemical irritation. This isn't serious; you can flush out the eyes with clean warm water.

What if one of my baby's eyes is always watering?

Excessive tearing is a very common problem in the first year of life, and is usually limited to one eye. Tears are normally secreted to keep the eye clean and moist, and drain from the eyes into the nose. In some babies, however, the tear-duct system fails to open completely, so that tears accumulate in the eyes. Your physician can show you how to massage the lacrimal sac and tear-duct system so the tears drain as they should.

Sometimes the eyes have a colored discharge as well, which may require a prescription of antibiotic drops. In most cases, massage and antibiotic drops will solve the problem. If persistent tearing continues until the child is twelve to fifteen months old, a relatively simple procedure of probing the tear duct can be carried out by an eye doctor.

When do babies start to see?

Babies can see at birth, though they don't have normal adult vision. Newborns can see large shapes—particularly faces, which have strong visual appeal. They appreciate strong, bright colors more readily than lighter shades. Visual development occurs very rapidly during the first year of life; by three months of age an infant will follow objects such as a ball or mobile in his or her line of vision. If your baby doesn't track objects in the visual field by this age, bring this to the doctor's attention.

What does it mean if my child's eyes are red?

A red or "bloodshot" eye is common, but should be checked by the doctor. Red eyes associated with tearing and itching, and particularly nasal congestion, indicate an allergic problem—often hay fever, asthma, or eczema. Treatment may include oral antihistamine-like medications or eye drops, or a combination of both.

A red or bloodshot eye may also be due to an infection, often contracted through contact with another child in the family or at the day-care center. Careful hand-washing is essential in treating these infections, as they are easily spread to the rest of the family.

Bacterial eye infections are usually associated with a discharge that is thick and yellow in color, and crusts the eyelid margins, particularly on awakening in the morning. This sort of infection is often accompanied by an upper-respiratory-tract infection. Treatment consists of bathing the eye in warm water, and sometimes oral antibiotics as well as antibiotic eye drops. Any child who has red eyes and significant yellow eye discharge should be assessed by a physician.

Often a viral infection causes "pink eye" and a prominent discharge, usually watery. Local lymph nodes may be swollen. Again the condition is highly infectious, and may spread through families and daycare centres. These viral infections are usually self-limiting, and no specific treatment is indicated, but your child's physician should be notified.

Whether the infection is thought to be bacterial or viral, a child with discharge from the eye should be kept away from other children to avoid spreading the condition.

A red eye can also be caused by inflammation of the eyelid (blepharitis), a condition involving the eyelashes and surrounding glands. This is often associated with a scaling skin condition such as seborrhea, or with a chronic bacterial infection of the eyelids. As the condition progresses there may be crusting and discharge, and the child may complain of itching in the eye. This type of infection is treated with local antibiotics.

Scaling skin around the eyes—often a greasy, dandruff-like scale on the lashes—may be associated with scaling of the scalp and ears. It's best treated by scrubbing the lid margins nightly for a month with a cotton swab and a non-irritating baby shampoo.

What if there's a boil on the eyelid?

This is a sty, a localized infection of the eyelid that also involves the surrounding glands. The whole eyelid is usually red, swollen, and tender. You can apply warm compresses for fifteen minutes four times a day, and a local antibiotic may be prescribed. A sty generally drains within a few days. If it persists for several weeks, your physician may refer you to an eye doctor.

Do red eyes ever indicate a serious problem?

More serious conditions are due to bacterial infection of the tissues surrounding the eye or eye socket. They are usually associated with a high fever; the child appears ill and there may be marked swelling or protrusion of the eye. The skin around the eye is red. These infections sometimes follow injury to the eye area, or a respiratory infection involving the sinuses, which are close to the eye. They must be assessed by a physician immediately, and appropriate antibiotic therapy must be given, usually in hospital.

A persistent red eye that is not associated with a discharge may indicate a more complicated eye problem, particularly if there is pain and sensitivity to light, or decreased vision. This calls for immediate attention from an eye specialist.

Should I worry if my baby's eyes seem crossed?

During well-baby visits, the physician will be checking to see that your baby's eyes are working together and that there is good sight in each eye. Though an infant's eyes may not be coordinated in the first few months of life, persistence of a "crossed" eye after the age of six months should be brought to the physician's attention, as should any family history of visual problems.

Crossed eyes, or strabismus, indicate that the eye muscles are not properly aligned, so that one eye deviates from its normal position. However, some children whose eyes appear crossed merely have a broad, flat nasal bridge, creating the illusion of crossed eyes. As the nose matures, this appearance goes away. Let the doctor decide whether your baby really has crossed eyes, or just a broad nasal ridge. If the eyes are crossed beyond six months of age, the condition will not go away without treatment by an eye doctor.

It's important to treat crossed eyes because the misalignment presents the brain with two different images. Since the brain has trouble processing these two images at the same time, it will gradually suppress the images from one eye, leading to a marked reduction in vision in that eye.

Crossed eyes can sometimes be corrected non-surgically, with eye patches and eyeglasses, but surgery may be required when non-surgical methods don't work.

When should my child's vision first be checked?

In addition to the checks done at well-baby visits in the first two years of life, a child's vision may be evaluated by three to four years of age. For example, the child may be shown a large letter E in various positions and taught to point his or her fingers in the same direction as the "fingers" of the E. This may require some advance practice with parents, so that the child feels ready to cooperate. Pictures are used as well, though this depends on the maturity of the child; some young patients don't cooperate because of lack of experience with the pictures, or an inability to name them.

Can't I wait to see if visual problems go away on their own?

Your child's psychological and learning development requires normal, coordinated vision. If visual defects aren't corrected early, development may be seriously impaired. Worse yet, there may be permanent damage to your child's vision.

Aren't there eye exercises to correct learning problems?

The use of exercises to compensate for specific learning and reading disabilities is not as yet supported by scientific evidence.

Ear Problems

Ear infections (otitis media) are the bacterial infections that most often bring children to the doctor in the first three years of life. Most occur between the ages of six months and two years, and children who have their first attack before the age of one are more likely to have recurrent infections than those who have their first bout later.

The anatomy of the ear

The ear has three main areas—outer (the ear canal we can see), middle (where sounds are transmitted from the eardrum by a delicate arrangement of bones), and inner (where sound signals are passed to the auditory nerve and the brain). The middle ear is connected to the throat by the eustachian tube. If the outside pressure changes (when we go up in an airplane, for example), the difference between outer-ear pressure and inner-ear pressure pushes on the eardrum, making us uncomfortable. Older children learn to "equalize" this pressure by yawning or swallowing to let air from the throat into the eustachian tubes; it's not so easy to manoeuvre infants into opening their eustachian tubes. Swelling or congestion of the eustachian tube can make equalization impossible, so that pressure differences create pain.

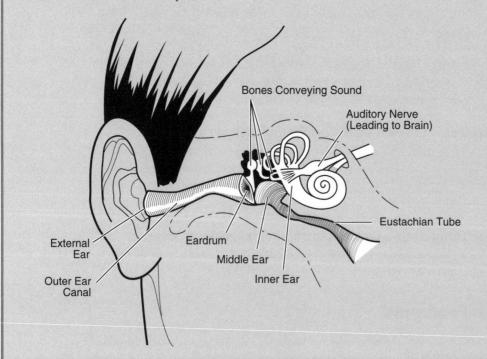

Bones Conveying Sound

Auditory Nerve
(Leading to Brain)

Eustachian Tube

External
Ear

Eardrum

Middle Ear

Inner Ear

Outer Ear
Canal

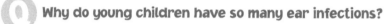

Why do young children have so many ear infections?

There are many contributing factors. Children in this age group have fairly low levels of protective antibodies, and increasing exposure to respiratory infections in day care and other gatherings. Their eustachian tubes are relatively short and have less supporting cartilage; the cartilage keeps the tube open because it is fairly rigid. With less cartilage, it's like a kinked hose. Any upper-respiratory-tract infection causes congestion of the lining of the respiratory tract and eustachian tube, making fluid accumulate in the middle ear. Germs proliferate in these secretions, and ear infections are the result.

Other factors, such as respiratory allergies and underlying anatomical defects (a cleft palate, for example), sometimes account for recurrent ear infections. Secondary cigarette smoke and excess humidity may be factors as well. (Cigarette smoke affects the protective lining of the eustachian tube so that bacteria can't easily be removed by the cells of the lining.)

It's true that infants and young children have relatively more lymphoid tissue, such as adenoids and tonsils, to protect the respiratory tract and help in the production of antibodies. However, these tissues—particularly the adenoids, when they're swollen—can obstruct the eustachian tube and further block drainage.

Does breast-feeding help prevent ear infections?

The role of breast-feeding in protecting against ear infections is somewhat controversial; so is the role of food allergies.

When are ear infections most likely?

Most occur during the "cold season," because of the frequency of respiratory infections at that time of year. Most ear infections are initiated by viral infections or mild upper-respiratory-tract infections (colds). Usually there is a slight fever and some nasal congestion, and the youngster becomes increasingly irritable and unhappy, sleeping and feeding poorly, and often developing a higher temperature. The fact that an infant pulls on his or her ear is not a reliable sign of an ear infection, but an older child will give verbal or other indications of pain in the affected ear. He or she should be seen by a physician, who will diagnose the ear infection by examining the child and observing the eardrum and its mobility.

It's sometimes very difficult to examine the eardrum of a young infant or child. Proper examination may be possible only after removing wax from the ear canal by careful syringing by the child's physician.

Treatment will be a ten-day course of an appropriate antibiotic, with follow-up by the physician in two weeks' time. The child's discomfort and fever can be treated with acetaminophen (such as Tempra or Tylenol). If the nose is badly blocked, a saline nose-drop preparation may help, or excess mucus may be aspirated (sucked out). The child should show improvement within forty-eight hours. If there is persistent fever or a worsening of the symptoms after that time, the child must be reassessed to be certain that the prescribed medication is appropriate, and that no more serious complication has developed.

 Are these antibiotics safe?

Some parents are reluctant to have their child on antibiotics, particularly for recurrent bouts of ear infections over a relatively long period of time. Remember that your doctor is very aware of the possible side effects of antibiotics; your child's medical history, particularly any previous allergy to a medication or any significant side effect, will be taken into account. And the benefits are substantial. Since the advent of antibiotic therapy, we no longer see the serious problems that were so prevalent only a few years ago: chronic mastoid infection, draining ears, and major hearing loss. Even life-threatening complications of ear infections, such as brain abscess and meningitis, have decreased significantly because of antibiotics.

 What happens once my child is on antibiotics?

By the follow-up examination two weeks later, there is usually marked improvement, although some fluid may remain in the middle ear. If this is the case, the physician will follow the child's progress over the next few months to be sure the fluid drains. If fluid is still present after three months, the child may need a hearing test to see whether the quantity of fluid is significant. If hearing is being affected, a long-term course of low-dose antibiotics may clear it up, avoiding the need for surgery.

 Can decongestants or antihistamines be used for middle-ear infections?

The use of oral nasal decongestants and antihistamines for these infections has not been shown to be effective. In addition, many of these medications cause side-effects such as drowsiness, excitability, and irritability, which make the child's condition more difficult to evaluate.

What happens if my child keeps getting ear infections?

Children who have frequent bouts of ear infection, particularly over the winter months, should be given a course of prophylactic (preventive) antibiotics. This approach is particularly effective in children aged six months to four years who have more than three bouts in a six-month period. These antibiotics are safe and inexpensive; just half the usual dose is given, once a day.

Children who keep getting ear infections even with prophylactic antibiotics may need surgery to drain the ears and insert ventilating tubes through the eardrum and into the middle ear. This is the commonest operation performed on children today, and is very safe, but it should be undertaken only after evaluation by the child's physician in consultation with an ear, nose, and throat specialist. They will consider not only the number of ear infections, but hearing problems, the persistence of thick fluid in the middle ear, reduced mobility of the eardrum, and persistent abnormal or negative pressure in the middle ear.

If tubes are inserted, they usually fall out or are removed after a few months, and the holes in the eardrum heal naturally.

About 10 percent of children later require a further set (or sets) of ventilating tubes. In this case, another course of prophylactic antibiotics should be considered, particularly over the winter, when respiratory infections are common.

Why all this fuss over an ear infection?

Children with ear infections are irritable and have a significant amount of pain. They need quick and efficient treatment to relieve their symptoms, and to keep the ear infection from leading to more serious problems. Also, an aggressive approach to the infection may keep the child from missing valuable time at school or daycare.

Some children with recurrent bouts of ear infection, and associated abnormalities of middle-ear pressure, exhibit behavioural changes. Whether their language and speech development suffers is less clear, although there is of course concern that significant hearing loss in both ears may account for some delay. There is as yet no agreement as to the minimum hearing sensitivity that infants and young children need for the complex process of developing speech and language successfully.

All children who have recurrent bouts of ear infection should be evaluated for middle-ear fluid. This can be done initially in the doctor's office, by observing the eardrum and evaluating middle-ear pressure by tympanometry (a technique using air pressure). Hearing evaluation by audiometry, using an electronic device that produces sounds for the child to hear, may also be necessary.

Are all ear infections in the middle ear?

Infections of the ear canal, commonly called "swimmer's ear," are often seen in the summer months. These can cause extreme pain, due to inflammation and the accumulation of debris in the ear canal. Treatment consists of painkillers, irrigation (flushing out) of the debris, and use of a combination ear drop containing antibiotics and cortisone.

What about other kinds of hearing problems?

Babies in high-risk groups—those with a family history of hearing loss or deafness, premature infants, and infants who need treatment in a neonatal intensive care unit—should be observed for possible hearing deficiency in the first few months of life.

Your own observations of your infant are very important in assessing his or her response to voices and general noise, and your intuitions are valuable. Any concerns you have about the baby's response to verbal or other stimulation should be brought to the attention of the physician.

Most toddlers have a vocabulary of about ten words by eighteen months and twice as many words by twenty-one months. By two years of age, most are linking a couple of words together. If your child is slow to reach these milestones, point this out to the doctor. A complete evaluation will include an ear, nose, and throat examination and a full assessment of the child's social and psychological background.

Toddlers who show delay in language development should have their hearing assessed by audiometry. Note, however, that infants from disadvantaged social situations or chaotic home environments may be delayed in language development. Some children who are constantly exposed to another language, perhaps from babysitters or grandparents, show a delay in language development, but they usually catch up by the age of four or five.

CHAPTER 12

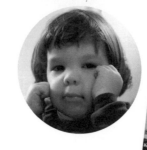

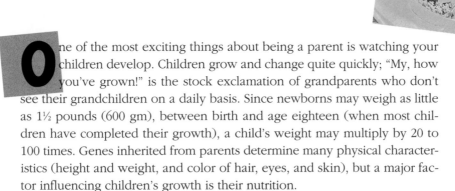

Feeding Your Child

One of the most exciting things about being a parent is watching your children develop. Children grow and change quite quickly; "My, how you've grown!" is the stock exclamation of grandparents who don't see their grandchildren on a daily basis. Since newborns may weigh as little as 1½ pounds (600 gm), between birth and age eighteen (when most children have completed their growth), a child's weight may multiply by 20 to 100 times. Genes inherited from parents determine many physical characteristics (height and weight, and color of hair, eyes, and skin), but a major factor influencing children's growth is their nutrition.

Obviously children need the right nutrients for growth, and to provide energy for daily activities. But they also need to acquire good eating habits, which will have a strong impact on their future food choices and health. Feeding infants and young children also helps them feel secure that they are loved. Feeding should be a time of happiness and pleasure, a time to promote love and security; it is not a time for speed, efficiency, or neatness. Food should be enjoyed!

How do I get my child to eat the right foods?

Although you should make sure your child gets a complete and well-balanced diet, you needn't be overly anxious or particular about what he or she eats. Children have a natural tendency to eat the right foods, in suitable amounts. Despite cultural diversity and varied ethnic traditions around the world, most societies have come up with appropriate diets. What an Inuit child in the Arctic and a vegetarian child in South Asia eat may be very different, but each diet may be ideally suited for the child in question. But keep in mind the fact that children learn by example. If you want your children to develop healthy, nutritious eating habits, you have to set an example.

115

Q **How do I know if I'm choosing the right foods?**

Our food can be considered in terms of carbohydrates, proteins, fats, vitamins, and minerals. Carbohydrates, in simple sugar forms or in complex starch forms, provide energy. Proteins are used to build and repair the body. Fats are used as more concentrated sources of energy, and to build certain body structures, such as the brain and nervous tissue. Vitamins (A, the B group, C, D, E, and K) and minerals (sodium, potassium, iron, calcium, magnesium, and others) are used in the normal growth and maintenance of our bodies. As a general rule, you don't have to worry about exactly what your child eats, as long as his or her diet accords with commonsense food guidelines, which suggest a reasonable balance of breads, cereals, and grains for energy; protein foods like meat, fish, or beans for body growth; fruits and vegetables for vitamins and minerals; and milk and dairy products for all these benefits. Most children who eat a balanced diet get adequate vitamins, so vitamin supplements are rarely appropriate for healthy children.

Feeding an Infant
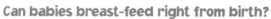

"Breast Is Best" is a slogan used by most pediatricians; all mothers should be encouraged to breast-feed. Breast milk is perfectly suited for the newborn, and—in spite of science and advertising—no other infant food is superior to human milk. It provides the ideal combination of essential proteins, fats, and carbohydrates for newborns, as well as some natural protection against infections. For the child with an inherited tendency to allergic reactions such as eczema or asthma, breast milk has fewer allergenic substances than cow's milk or soy-based formula (although there is little solid evidence that breast-feeding actually protects infants from such allergic conditions). Finally, breast-feeding encourages bonding between mother and child, helps mothers understand the cues infants give regarding their needs, and can be very convenient for both mother and child. It's also inexpensive.

Q **Can babies breast-feed right from birth?**

During the first week, breast-feeding may not be easy. Very little breast milk is produced in the first two days. Also, it may be difficult for a newborn to latch on to the mother's breast, and some mothers find it uncomfortable. It's important to get prenatal and postnatal teaching and hands-on help from the nurse in the hospital, and a nurse, physician, or midwife during the first few weeks at home. In 1996 the in-hospital rate for woman who breast-fed their newborns was 59.2 percent.

If they are supported and encouraged by their families, friends, and physicians, most mothers will be able to breast-feed. If they have difficulty, they can seek advice from public-health nurses, family physicians or pediatricians, or lactation consultants. Once breast-feeding is established, most mothers feed their children "on demand," usually every two to four hours.

Do breast-feeding babies need extra vitamins and minerals?

Some experts are not convinced that infants in our northern climates get enough vitamin D. Vitamin D is normally produced in people by sunlight, and is added to commercial cow's milk. A deficiency of vitamin D results in a disease called "rickets" (weakened bones). Rickets used to be common, but is now rarely seen because of vitamin D supplements. If lactating mothers have an adequate source of vitamin D, and if they and their children are outdoors in the sunshine, there's no need for supplements. But during the winter months, when mothers and children tend to remain indoors, they may not get enough vitamin D. Although there is evidence that most lactating mothers produce adequate amounts of the vitamin for the first six months, many authorities recommend vitamin D supplements for breast-feeding infants. They are readily available in the form of drops in drugstores.

Fluoride is important for developing teeth, and adding fluoride to the water supply in most communities has resulted in a lower rate of children's dental cavities. If your water supply is low in fluoride, you should give your breast-fed infant fluoride in liquid form, using a dropper. Note that, as with most substances, too much can create a problem. Excess fluoride can cause tooth discoloring called "fluorosis." You should discuss the need for fluoride supplements with your physician or public-health nurse.

Your physician will also give you advice about iron supplements. Breast milk has little iron, but the iron in it is much more readily absorbed than other forms of iron in food. For the first six months of life, there is enough iron in breast milk to allow for normal growth and normal production of red blood cells. However, some newborns—especially premature and low-birthweight infants—have only a small amount of iron stored in their bodies, and require iron supplements. By four to six months of age, most children should be started on solid foods that contain iron. In North America this usually means prepared infant cereals, which are fortified with iron. Other good sources of iron include meats, green vegetables, eggs, and iron-fortified breads.

117

Hints on breast-feeding

- Breast-milk production does not "turn on" until the third or fourth day, but during this interval a small amount of fluid called "colostrum," high in energy and antibodies, is flowing. The newborn doesn't need a lot of fluid; there is an excess in the tissues at birth, which is why most babies lose up to 10 percent of their birthweight in the first two or three days of life.

- Not all babies learn immediately to "latch on" to the breast. Some authorities feel that giving bottles, or even pacifiers, too early can cause further confusion.

- In the early days or weeks it's best to feed "on demand" (but at least every four or five hours). With time, the frequency of feeding will naturally decrease from every two hours to every four. By six months of age, your baby will likely be sleeping eight to ten hours at night.

- When feeding or crying, babies may swallow lots of air. Most of it passes into the bowel and is absorbed. Some may remain in the stomach, taking up space and making your baby feel full. Burping after feeding from the first breast is helpful, but you should persist for only two or three minutes before carrying on with the feed.

- Unlimited suckling from the beginning has been shown to improve the success rate of breast-feeding, and does not lead to sore nipples. Sore nipples are usually from improper positioning of the infant on the breast. The baby should suck on the dark portion of the breast (the areola) behind the nipple.

- The baby will empty the breast in six to eight minutes. The highest fat content of breast milk is in the last portion of the feeding. Try feeding the baby ten minutes on one side, burping the baby, then nursing for ten to fifteen minutes on the other side.

- In the early stages there may be more milk than the baby needs. This may be a good time to pump the excess and store it in the freezer; it can be stored for up to six months. Do not thaw it in the microwave!

- A baby wets six to eight diapers per day if he or she is getting enough milk. With the new super-absorbent diapers it's sometimes difficult to assess the urine output. Hold a fresh diaper in one hand and the used diaper in the other and compare the weights.

- The occasional baby who is not obtaining enough nutrition from the breast can be given supplements, without resorting to the bottle, by various means including "lactation aids," finger feeding, or a cup. These techniques have to be taught by breast-feeding consultants. There is recent evidence, however, that a bottle or two per day does *not* lead to "nipple confusion."

Are there reasons not to breast-feed?

Some women prefer not to breast-feed because of previous negative experience, personal feelings, breast surgery, etc. Others who are ill or have nipple abnormalities have difficulties breast-feeding. If you are taking medications on a regular basis, discuss this with your doctor; most medications, including alcohol and nicotine, pass into the breast milk. If you are on hormones, or drugs for cancer, thyroid disease, or certain psychiatric illnesses, you may be advised not to breast-feed.

How long should babies breast-feed?

According to the La Leche League, only 21.7 percent of the 59.2 percent of women who breast-fed their infants in hospital continued to do so after six months. Ideally it may be best to continue until the child is about a year old and can go from breast-feeding to regular cow's milk in a cup.

What's in that formula?

In general, formulas fall into four categories:

- cow's milk as the base

- soya beans as the base

- cow's milk as the base, with the sugar changed so it doesn't contain lactose

- hydrolysed casein/whey formula, with the protein broken down into smaller pieces less likely to cause an allergic reaction

---

What about bottle-fed babies?

If you choose to bottle-feed, you needn't feel guilty about it; today's commercial formulas are designed to approximate the composition of breast milk, and most children thrive and develop just as well on formula. Formula uses cow's milk or soy protein as a base but is modified to be lower in protein than cow's milk and to contain all the necessary vitamins and minerals. In spite of advertisements, there is very little difference between the various brands of formula, except for those prepared specifically for premature infants. Most physicians and nutritionists recommend an iron-fortified formula. Products are generally available in three forms: ready-to-use, which is the most expensive; as a concentrated liquid, to be diluted; or as a powder which is added to water. Be sure you prepare the formula exactly according to the manufacturer's instructions. Most infants take at least 2 to 3 ounces per pound (150 to 180 mL per kilo) of formula each day. A baby four to six months old who gets most nutrition from milk formula may take a maximum of about 34 ounces (1200 mL) per day. However, after six months of age children start to get their daily nutrients from other foods and usually take much less milk. Infant formula should be used for about nine months, and then you can introduce homogenized cow's milk. An older baby who consumes too much milk or dairy products will be missing out on other foods, which could lead to dietary imbalance and possibly iron-deficiency anemia.

How do I make sure my baby's bottles are sterile?

In the past most parents were careful about sterilizing milk before giving it to their children, but the techniques they used may not be necessary. It is important, however, to wash your hands carefully before making up formula, and to use bottles, nipples, and water that are clean and germ-free. Although many parents boil the bottles and nipples, evidence suggests that fewer than 50 percent manage to prepare sterile formula. By four to six months of age, when children are putting everything in their mouths anyway, it may just be important to use clean bottles. Most parents make up one day's supply of milk and keep the bottles in the refrigerator. Most infants take formula more readily if it's warmed, although there is little evidence that they prefer it this way. Be wary of overheating formula in a microwave oven; always test the temperature before giving it to your child. Never put an infant to bed with a propped-up bottle, as the child may choke or inhale the milk; also, the constant presence of milk in the mouth encourages the growth of bacteria, producing acid and cavities.

Why are some babies put on soy-based formula?

Soy formula is used for babies with either a milk allergy or a lactose intolerance. A *milk allergy* is a reaction to the protein in cow's milk; it may show up as a rash, coughing or wheezing, diarrhea, or colic (see Chapter 4, "Crying"). These symptoms should go away when the child is taken off cow's milk.

A *lactose intolerance* is a deficiency of lactase, the enzyme that breaks down the sugar in milk (lactose). Some children inherit a lactase deficiency; others develop it temporarily after a severe bout of gastroenteritis (intestinal flu). The problem shows up as continued diarrhea, or bloating, gas, and abdominal pain. These problems should go away when the child is taken off cow's milk products (soy does not contain lactose).

Lactose intolerance is more common in certain ethnic groups, notably blacks and orientals. However, it tends to be overdiagnosed; it's important to see if the symptoms actually stop completely when milk is removed from the diet, and recur when milk is reintroduced. Your doctor can arrange for a specific test (a breath hydrogen test) if there is any doubt about the diagnosis.

Note that the soy-based drinks sold in many grocery and health-food stores do not have the same nutrients as formula, and should not be given to infants in place of formula.

Can I give my baby low-fat milk?

During the first year of life, a child needs fats for normal growth of the brain and nervous system, and should be given only *full-fat* milk formula—not 2 percent or skim milk. Note also that goat's milk, which is low in vitamins and folic acid, is a poor choice for infants, and that unpasteurized (raw) milk could lead to serious intestinal infections and a deficiency of vitamin D, and should never be used.

When can I start giving my baby other foods?

Newborn infants need only breast milk or formula. By three to six months, babies may be offered juice diluted half and half with water, or juices specifically prepared for infants. (Since breast milk and formula both contain vitamin C, the juice is offered only for the sake of variety.) Be sure juices don't replace other foods in your baby's diet. An infant should have no more than 4 ounces (125 mL) per day, a child over eighteen months no more than 8 ounces (250 mL) a day. On hot days, when they lose more water by sweating—or when they are dehydrated by diarrhea—they may take extra water between feedings. As children grow older and can indicate their thirst, they should be encouraged to drink water so they don't get into the habit of drinking too much juice or pop.

By four to six months of age, most infants have started infant cereals. Start with single-grain cereals with added iron, such as rice cereal. Barley, oat, or wheat can be tried later. The cereals are usually made with a small amount of breast milk or warmed cow's milk or water, and offered twice a day. Most parents start with a small spoonful or two, and let their children decide how much to take. Often parents offer half the breast- or formula-feeding before the cereal, and then complete the feeding after the child has had as much cereal as he or she wants.

Offering cereal before four months of age is neither necessary nor very successful. The natural movement of the newborn's tongue is up and forward to compress the nipple, which tends to push out solid food. It's about three or four months before infants can push food to the back of the mouth to be swallowed.

Baby teeth start to erupt around six months of age, and by that time infants are ready to eat strained or puréed foods. You can buy these in small jars, or make your own with a blender; home-prepared purées are equally nutritious, and cheaper. There's no need to add salt to infant foods as you might to your own.

There are few rigid rules for introducing infant foods. Cereals, fortified with iron, should probably be introduced first, but then see what your infant likes. Children have some sense of taste but appear to be less concerned about flavors than adults are. Respect your child's likes and dislikes, but encourage the sampling of many foods so he or she learns to eat a variety. Begin with bland, non-allergenic foods. Most parents start with vegetables (puréed carrots, squash, sweet or white potatoes, beans), and later add fruits (bananas, apples, peaches, and pears) and meats (chicken, lamb). It's important to introduce only one new food at a time, and wait for three or four days before introducing another. That way, if your child has an allergic reaction (a rash, diarrhea, or vomiting), you can more easily identify the offending food.

Yellow or orange vegetables (carrots, squash), which are frequently given to infants, may add a yellowish tinge to the skin, including the palms of the hands and the soles of the feet, but not to the eyes. This phenomenon is called "carotenemia" and is caused by the carotene in these vegetables; it has no significance and does no harm to the child.

By one year of age most children show an interest in a cup and can be weaned from the bottle. A cup, particularly one with a spout and two handles, enables the child to feed without help.

 ## Do babies need fiber to avoid constipation?

Breast-fed infants may have infrequent stools, because breast milk is almost completely absorbed, but their stools are soft and not painful to pass; this is not constipation. On the other hand, formula-fed infants who take few solids with any fiber may be constipated, with small, pellet-like, and occasionally blood-streaked painful stools. Once children start eating more foods, make sure they get some containing fiber, including diluted prune juice, fruits, vegetables, and whole-wheat breads and cereals.

From six months of age on, about one tooth per month erupts, until all twenty have appeared by about the age of two. During this period, when the teeth are appearing and children have more hand control, they like to put things in their mouths and chew them. You can offer soft biscuits or bread to let them feed themselves, but it's not until about one year of age that they have enough teeth to really chew. After that point they can be offered junior foods or soft cooked foods that require some chewing. At this stage they want their independence; encourage them to feed themselves, no matter how messy this gets. They also develop more likes and dislikes, and some become picky eaters. There's no need to worry if your child doesn't eat at some meals; what matters is how much he or she eats over several days. This is best demonstrated by the child's ongoing weight gain.

 How often should children be fed?

Most mothers who breast-feed do so whenever the child seems hungry. Most premature infants are fed every one to three hours, and full-term infants every two to four hours (six feedings a day). By the time children are sleeping through the night, they usually get five feedings a day. When solids are first introduced, they are given once or twice a day. By one year of age, most children are on three meals a day, with two or three snacks between mealtimes. Endless snacking; sugary, high-fat items; and excessive quantities of juice or pop should be discouraged. Children should be taught to eat when hungry and stop when satisfied.

Feeding an Older Child
....

In the past, physicians often gave parents strict rules about what and how much to feed their children. In most cases these rules are unnecessary; children eat according to their needs, and it's more important to offer them a balance of foods, avoiding too much added sugar, coloring, and flavor. The 1980s and 1990s have seen a return to simpler, more traditional, less-processed foods. Some childhood problems, such as dental cavities from too much refined sugar or constipation from a lack of dietary fiber, may be avoided by using these more basic foods.

Some foods are dangerous because they can get stuck in the child's windpipe (trachea) or esophagus (food passage). Hot dogs, grapes, and carrots are all the right size and shape to get stuck. For young children, hot dogs or grapes should be sliced in half or cut in small pieces. Peanuts (even crunchy peanut butter) and raw, hard, uncooked vegetables or fruit should not be offered to children under four, for the same reason.

Introducing solids

1. Introduce cereals somewhere between four and six months of age.

2. Start with rice cereal the first week (it's hypoallergenic). Offer it to your baby in small amounts (less than a tablespoon) twice daily. Use a small, soft infant spoon.

3. In the second week try a new cereal, such as oatmeal, once daily, again in small amounts. Give rice at a second feeding, in whatever quantity your baby craves.

4. In the third week introduce another new cereal, perhaps barley or soya. As before, the new food should be given in small amounts each day. The previously tried cereals can be given at a second meal in amounts that seem to satisfy your child. Avoid mixed cereal initially as it contains wheat, which is a little more allergenic.

5. Now it's time for vegetables. They are palatable, colorful, and less sweet than fruits. Besides, you won't kick yourself for creating a sweet tooth when your youngster turns off vegetables later on. Again, begin with a small amount given daily, as a third meal (e.g., lunch) or as part of another feeding. Previously tried cereals may be given at the same time.

6. Start with the yellow vegetables, such as squash, sweet potato, or carrots. They are less likely to cause gas than beans, and are less allergenic than legumes such as peas. Again, try one new food at a time, about a week apart. Give it daily, alone or with other foods that your baby seems to like. Commercial preparations are quite acceptable.

 What if allergies run in the family?

If your family has a history of allergic diseases (eczema, hay fever, asthma, or food allergies), it's wise to avoid the more commonly allergenic foods. Food allergies are a greater problem for infants under one year old, since their digestive tracts allow small amounts of allergenic foods to cross the lining of the intestinal tract unchanged. If possible, breast-feed for at least a year. Delay the introduction of potentially allergenic solids such as eggs and wheat. Some children are allergic to the soy-based formulas used for children with a milk allergy; they may need hydrolysed casein/whey formula. Children under one year of age shouldn't be given egg white, although they may have egg yolk. Just because you have a particular food allergy doesn't mean your children will have the same one, so you needn't withhold the food in question; just watch closely for any indications of an allergic reaction.

Introducing solids (continued)

7. Next comes fruit, one kind at a time. Pears and peaches tend to soften stools, whereas bananas and apples firm them up. Avoid citrus fruits at this early stage as they are more likely to cause a reaction.

8. Apple juice may be started along with applesauce. It's excessively sweet, so dilute it with approximately three parts water to each part juice. Limit the quantity, except on sweltering days. Juice, like formula, does not belong in a crib.

9. After three or four different fruits, you can try meats. Don't be surprised if your baby baulks at them; how crazy are you about boiled beef? Start with chicken, then try turkey or veal. Hard-boiled egg yolk (not white) can be given next, but only once or twice weekly.

10. Table foods are introduced at eight or nine months. Children (or their parents) seem ready to begin them at varying times. Whenever you start, choose foods your child can't choke on. Consider a peeled banana first. Partially puréed cooked vegetables can also be started. Use fresh or frozen foods rather than canned. You can then try short pasta—it's hard to choke on a noodle. Bagels and bread-crust are good to gnaw on. Stewed soft meats and boneless fish such as tuna or fishsticks are the best way to initiate this food group. Avoid extra salt and excessive sweetening of table foods. Let children enjoy each food's natural taste.

11. Finally, take the time to really enjoy feeding your child. In our hectic world, few things are more important or fulfilling than a good meal with your loved ones.

How can I be sure if my child has food allergies?

Many families get caught up in a pattern of avoiding all suspected foods, with the result that their children miss out on important nutrition such as calcium from milk, or iron. A child who suffers from an allergy will develop symptoms almost immediately after eating the problem food. Symptoms may be a rash, swelling of the lips, or difficulty breathing, or the diarrhea and gas associated with cow's-milk allergy. The most common food allergens are probably milk, peanuts and other legumes, fish and shellfish, and strawberries. Skin tests by an allergist will tell you what your child's *skin* reacts to, but this doesn't mean the child will react to *eating* the food. Most food allergies are diagnosed by the symptoms the child suffers after eating that food.

Making mealtimes work

Nutrition and Growth

- Children don't like to sit still, but they should be encouraged to stay in a highchair or at the table. This encourages them to concentrate on eating, and prevents injuries that may happen if a child falls while eating and running.

- Watch for signs that your child is full, such as turning away from a spoon or clamping the mouth shut. Don't hover expectantly while an older child eats. Children usually eat as much as they need to keep them going, even if the amount seems small.

- Never force or bribe a child to eat; children know when they're no longer hungry. When you introduce a new food, the child may resist and turn away; rather than insisting, try again later in the meal.

- Don't use food as a reward; the impression that food equals love or approval can contribute to later eating disorders. Food also shouldn't be used as a bribe for good behavior. Good behavior should be expected, and food, snacks, and treats should be a normal part of life.

- Offer only small amounts of food and fluids at a time. There's always more.

- Serve meals with a variety of tastes, colors, and textures, to make them more appealing. Give your child his or her own chair and place-setting, perhaps with colorful bowls and utensils.

- Remember that mood is catching. Mealtimes should be not just for eating, but for socializing with the family. Watching TV is a poor substitute for family interaction.

- Don't "hurry along" meals. Allow young children time for play and experimentation, but stop before the mess becomes too annoying. A stress-free atmosphere promotes good lifetime food attitudes.

- Ignore food-throwing at first; it's part of normal development. Children drop things to learn the "letting go" reflex, and how better to practise than by dumping bits of food from a highchair? Clean-up will be easier if you put newspaper or plastic sheets under the highchair. But once your child acquires the skill of letting go, don't encourage this "game" by continually picking up dropped food. Instead, after a few throws, remove the food—the child is likely full.

- Encourage independence. Children need to practice eating, and success helps them feel good about themselves.

- Let toddlers pick food from the serving plate so they feel free to choose what and how much to eat. This helps reduce frustration during the "no" stage. Providing limited and realistic choices encourages children to think independently. Encourage eating with a spoon so your child learns to handle utensils, but allow some finger foods to smooth the transition.

Can the baby share our family's vegetarian diet?

Many children in this world are raised on vegetarian diets, sometimes including milk (lacto-vegetarian) or eggs (ovo-vegetarian). A true "vegan" diet, which avoids meat, milk, and eggs, can be dangerous for young children as there may be a deficiency of iron, calcium, or vitamin B_{12}. Note that a vegetarian diet shouldn't consist only of the avoidance of meat; vegetable proteins don't always have all the essential amino acids, and you may need to serve foods in specific combinations to create a complete nutritional package. Families with a long tradition of vegetarian diets, for cultural or religious reasons, know how to provide all the important dietary requirements for their children, but families just starting on a vegetarian diet are advised to read books or talk with a dietitian about providing balanced nutrition.

What can I do about a child who just won't eat?

Most children have good and bad days for eating. Many have favorite foods and are reluctant to eat anything else. These food preferences come and go, as long as you don't "give in" by offering nothing but the favorites.

But a few children refuse to take any food, turning their faces away, clamping their mouths shut when food is offered, or spitting out any food you get into them. On rare occasions this is due to a physical problem, such as pain from stomach acid coming back up into the lower end of the esophagus. More often, it's learned behavior. Some children just don't want to eat as much as their parents would like them to, so they turn stubborn and resist whatever is offered. Children who are force-fed may find the experience painful, and refuse to cooperate. Others learn that when they refuse to eat they get more attention. The reasons for the behavior are often complicated, but the response of the parent is generally to try to force the child to eat. *You can't force children to eat more, but you can make sure you offer foods high in calories.* There are some simple guidelines to help persuade a picky eater into having a good meal.

- Meals should be well prepared, appetizing, and the kind of food the child likes, though it's not necessary to give in to every want or demand. New foods should be added gradually, in small amounts, along with food your child knows and likes. Mealtimes should be planned for times when the child is hungry. Having a child wait may disrupt his or her normal appetite.

- Offer three meals and three snacks a day, and don't offer food at other times. Nibbling or drinking between meals just spoils the appetite. Some families spend the whole day trying to get their children to eat, and then wonder why the child isn't hungry at mealtime! Snacks should be nutritious foods—fruits, vegetables, crackers and cheese or peanut butter—not a lot of candies, cakes, and cookies.

- If your child doesn't eat within a given time, such as twenty or thirty minutes, the food should be put away and nothing else offered until the next meal or snack. If your child doesn't eat what you've prepared, don't prepare something else more to his or her liking.

- Take along extra milk or a snack on your child's excursions. Find time for a healthy snack when you're out, just as you would at home.

Q What if my child doesn't seem to be growing?

Children usually double their birthweight in the first four or five months and triple it by one year. Then their growth levels off, and many parents worry that their children don't seem to be growing to the same extent, or eating as much.

Your child's growth should be followed on a regular basis by the child's physician, who will measure length or height and head circumference at each visit, comparing these with standards on a growth chart. Children should be weighed without clothes, or with diapers, on a good standardized scale. Under two years of age, length is measured lying down; after two years, standing height is measured.

The growth charts show the average weight and length/height for children at different ages, and the normal range expressed as from the 3rd to the 97th percentile. The charts were compiled by measuring healthy children in either London, England, or Boston, U.S.A., and they don't necessarily apply to children from other parts of the world. As well, children usually follow the growth pattern of their parents. If the parents are tall, the child will usually be above the halfway mark (50th percentile); if the parents are short, the child's height and weight will usually be below that line. Still, whatever the family background, a child's growth should *parallel* the pattern of the growth charts.

If a child's growth is not as expected, you should discuss this with the doctor, who will want to know the height and weight of both parents and their growth patterns. Some people are small throughout childhood and go into puberty later than their peers, but then have a delayed growth spurt and reach average adult size. This very common pattern of temporary smallness can be passed on to children, and causes a lot of unnecessary worry for parents.

Your physician will also ask about your child's health and eating, and will carry out a thorough physical exam. In most cases this will be enough to pinpoint the cause of your child's poor growth, without a lot of laboratory tests.

When children don't gain weight, it's most often because they don't eat enough good, nutritious food. The doctor can advise you on a better diet, but there's no "magic pill" to get a child to eat. No medication has been found to stimulate children's appetite on a long-term basis. If your child doesn't eat a well-balanced diet, a supplemental vitamin may be helpful. For children who are very thin and need to gain weight, there are supplemental foods that should be given only on the advice of your physician.

There are also a few simple things you can do to help your child gain weight. They depend on your child's age.

- For young infants, whose diets consist primarily of formula and/or puréed foods, you can fortify the foods with supplements. The formula can be concentrated by adding less water, but major changes in formula preparation should be done only with the advice of your physician or a good nutritionist.

- For toddlers and older children, prepare foods that are higher in calories, and at the same time help them improve their eating behavior.

- Fats are generally higher in calories than carbohydrates or proteins, so children who need to gain weight should be given higher-fat foods such as homogenized milk rather than 2 percent or skim, butter or margarine, cheese, cream, and peanut butter. Butter, margarine, salad oils and dressings, yogurt, sour cream, or cheese sauces can be added to other foods. But sweets such as candies, cakes, and cookies may satisfy children sooner than more nutritious complex-carbohydrate food such as starches, bread, pastas, potatoes, rice, or other cereals, so that in the end they eat *less*.

- Try making sandwiches with two slices of meat plus cheese; adding small pieces of cooked meat, poultry, or tofu to macaroni, omelettes, quiches, soups, or salads; spreading peanut butter on sandwiches, muffins, crackers, or pancakes; and serving nuts or seeds as snacks or added to ice cream or yogurt. (Nuts should not be given to children under four as they may accidentally go into the lungs.)

Overweight Children

Infants and toddlers have different body proportions than adults, with larger trunks and shorter legs. They may thus appear to be fat or "chubby" when they are normal, healthy children. However, some children do gain too much weight for their age and height. There is good evidence that obesity tends to run in families, both because of genetic factors and because children learn patterns of overeating and underexercising from their families.

Obesity is seen most commonly in one-year-olds, preschoolers, and young adolescents. It's usually the result of two factors: the children eat more than necessary, and are less active and don't burn off the calories they take in. If a child has a tendency to obesity, it's easier to deal with it early, before the child is grossly overweight. Weight-loss programs for children have generally been very unsuccessful unless the *child* is highly motivated to lose weight.

If you feel your infant or toddler is overweight, talk to the doctor before making major changes in the child's diet, to be certain the child is truly over-weight according to the growth chart; he or she may not be overweight at all. You have more control over what your child eats at this age, so you can help your child develop a diet that doesn't include high-calorie foods. (Initially this may be more useful than trying to control the *amount* the child eats.) After one year of age, overweight children should be given 2 percent rather than homogenized milk, smaller amounts of food, and foods with lower fat content.

There is little evidence that obesity in young children predisposes them to obesity in adulthood. There is also little evidence that early obesity predisposes children to weight-related diseases such as atherosclerosis (hardening of the arteries), heart disease, or diabetes in adulthood. On the other hand, we know that these diseases also tend to run in families. If your family has a history of obesity and these related conditions, it's prudent to try to manage your child's weight problem as early as possible.

 What about an older overweight child?
Avoid offering more food than the child wants, and don't offer food outside of regular meal and snack times. Snacks should be nutritious vegetables, fruits, crackers or breads. Juice, pop with sugar, and milk can provide a lot of calories; offer them in moderation. A child who is just thirsty should be given water.

Discourage your child from eating too much just before bedtime, which can set up bad habits. If physical activity and exercise are a normal pattern for your family, your child will readily copy your example.

If an older child is concerned about actual overweight, it may be best for the child to set the goal of maintaining present weight. As the child grows taller, the weight will be more appropriately distributed, with less fat. If the child wants to maintain weight, or even lose weight, it's probably best to encourage smaller amounts of low-fat foods rather than follow a specific weight-loss diet designed for adults. Children should avoid overeating, second helpings, eating when they're bored rather than hungry, and eating after supper. They should eat low-calorie foods, drink skim or 1 percent milk, and avoid excessive amounts of cheese, peanuts and peanut butter, fried and fatty foods, and french fries and chips. Snacks should be nutritious but low in calories: fruits and vegetables, popcorn without butter or margarine. Cakes and cookies should be avoided.

A child who wants to lose weight can benefit from regular walking with Mom or Dad or the dog, swimming, bicycling, skating, or skiing. Twenty to thirty minutes of exercise a day will burn up more calories than reading or watching television. Probably the activity that has contributed most to obesity in children is watching television, with snacks of chips or cookies close at hand.

What about an overweight teenager?

As children get into their teens, their behavior—including eating—is often influenced more by their peers and by advertising than by their parents. They want to "follow the crowd" and do what their friends do. For girls who are self-conscious about their weight, this may mean skipping meals, avoiding certain foods, or experimenting with diets. For boys who are concerned about their athletic ability, this may mean taking food, protein, or vitamin and mineral supplements. Some teens, especially those who are concerned about their weight or have a busy schedule, start to skip meals, particularly breakfast. Children need food energy for the day's activities. Breakfast is probably the most important meal, and should not be skipped.

Some teenagers stop drinking milk, or stop eating meat. Milk is a major source of calcium and vitamin D, required for bone growth, and is very important during puberty. Meat provides a valuable source of protein, vitamins, and iron. Inadequate intakes of calcium and iron are not uncommon in young people today. If your teenager wants to avoid certain foods, he or she should seek advice from a nutritionist or your physician.

Teenagers also spend a lot of time watching television and eating snacks. Again, it's not easy to tell them how to behave, but even teens tend to follow their parents' example.

As a parent, you need to be aware of what your child is or is not eating. It's pointless to force or nag or tell teens what to do, but you can help them seek good nutritional advice from your doctor, from magazines and books, or from nutritional counselors. Remember, bad eating habits are easier to prevent than to correct. You can help your children get off to a good start by showing them moderate, balanced eating habits, and a healthy lifestyle with regular exercise.

131

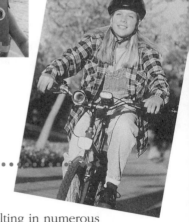

CHAPTER 13

Safety at Home and Away

I njuries are a leading health problem of children, resulting in numerous deaths and hospitalizations per year among children younger than fifteen years of age. More than half of all childhood deaths result from injuries, exceeding deaths due to cancer; congenital anomalies (problems present at birth); and diseases of the nervous system, heart, and respiratory system. Deaths are only the tip of the iceberg. It is estimated that for every injury death, more than 50 children are admitted to hospital, and 1,300 are treated in the emergency department.

Suffocation and choking are the leading causes of injury death for infants under one year, accounting for one-third of the total. The leading cause of injury hospitalization for infants is falls.

Motor vehicle collisions are the leading cause of injury death for children aged one to fourteen. Approximately half of these are pedestrian deaths, and about one-fifth of the school-age children who die in collisions are bicyclists. The leading cause of injury hospitalization for this age group, as for infants, is falls. After one year of age, boys suffer more of almost every kind of injury than girls.

Often these injuries are described as "accidents," which suggests that the harm could not have been expected, and therefore could not have been prevented. The more we understand about how injuries happen, the more we recognize that there are recurring patterns that *can* be anticipated, and changed. We should abandon the word "accident" and begin to consider most injuries *preventable*.

Q How can I predict what might happen to my child?

There are many factors that make a child vulnerable to one kind of injury or another. One is the child's temperament; impulsive, highly active children—

those sometimes called "accident-prone"—may be more at risk. Another is the child's development in various respects. A child in a normal independence-seeking phase may imitate risky behaviors; a child may or may not have the physical capabilities to cope with a particular kind of danger. Yet another is the environment, both physical and social; a child living by a river faces a different balance of risks than a child with an inattentive babysitter. All these factors are likely known or suspected by the parents; too often, not enough precautions are taken in spite of that knowledge.

What should I be doing about these risks?

There are a lot of steps parents can take on their own: supervising children more closely, "childproofing" homes, staying aware of the latest safety developments, and generally thinking ahead to the risks their children may encounter.

There are also steps that require the involvement of others. Some are technological; parental groups can press for more effective safety equipment, such as bicycle helmets and child car seats. Others are community concerns. Are there dangerous sites in your neighborhood that attract daredevil children? Should there be a stoplight at a certain intersection, or more spotchecks for drinking drivers? Consider what happens after an injury occurs. Are your fire and ambulance services well equipped? Could volunteers be trained for community emergencies? Does your local hospital need better facilities? You may want to get involved in a parents' coalition to tackle questions like these.

Motor Vehicle Collisions

How can I protect my child in a car crash?

Motor vehicle occupant injuries are the leading cause of death for older children and adolescents, and a common cause of death for children at younger ages. Fatal injuries are most often to the head, and brain, spinal cord, and facial injuries are frequent serious non-fatal injuries. These usually result when a child with no seatbelt or car safety seat is thrown against the interior of the car, such as the windshield, dashboard, or front seat.

Such "unrestrained" children are five to six times more likely to die in a motor vehicle crash than restrained children. Infants held in arms are as likely to be seriously injured or killed as unrestrained children; in a crash, it's physically impossible for an adult to hold on to an infant.

Car restraint devices do more than secure children to the car so they are less likely to hit the inside. They also spread the forces of the crash over the strongest parts of the child's body. But they must be installed following the manufacturer's guidelines. Incorrect installation is a very common problem, and decreases the child's protection. The ideal position for a child car seat is the center of the back seat. After purchasing a new car seat, remember to send in the registration form so the manufacturer can notify you of any problems with the seat.

The right type of car restraint for your child will change as the child grows. Don't be in a hurry to transfer your child from one device to the next, but follow the guidelines below so you'll know when your child has outgrown the old car seat.

Infants (0–9 months, under 20 lbs/9 kg)

Start using an infant car seat on the first ride home from the hospital; newborns are much safer in a properly installed infant seat than in a parent's arms. They should be placed in a rear-facing infant seat, or in a convertible seat in the rear-facing position. This has been designed especially for infants, who are small in size, with large heads and poor neck-muscle control and prominent tummies, and are unable to sit. The rear-facing design allows the force of a crash to be spread evenly across the whole body, pushing the baby's head and chest against the padded back of the seat. The car seatbelt should be pulled through the correct path on the infant seat and pulled tight. If the lap/shoulder belt doesn't stay tight (i.e., is not self-locking), check the car-seat instructions about using a metal locking clip. The harness should fit snugly over the infant's shoulders and between the legs. The plastic harness clip should be pulled up to armpit level to keep the straps on the shoulders; if not, the infant may be thrown out of the seat in the event of a crash. If the car is equipped with a front passenger-side airbag, the infant seat should be placed in the back seat. If the airbag inflates, it may cause serious injuries to a rear-facing infant in the front seat.

Toddlers and preschoolers (9 months to 4–5 years, 20 to 40 lbs/9 to 18 kg)

The rear-facing position is the safest way to travel at any age, but when an infant is at least 20 pounds (9 kg) and is able to sit unsupported he or she may be placed in a front-facing car seat, or the convertible seat can be turned

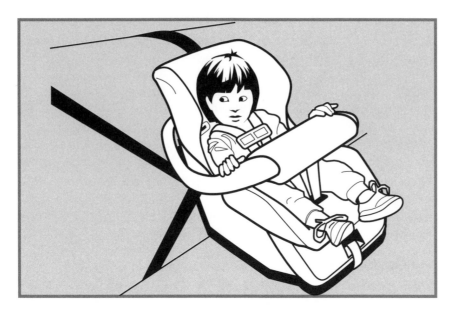

around to the forward-facing position. The harness straps and shield spread the force of a crash over the strongest parts of the body—that is, the shoulders and hips, instead of the neck and abdomen. Again, the car seatbelt should be pulled through correctly and pulled tight to keep the base of the safety seat in place, and if the seatbelt doesn't stay tight you should check the instructions about using a metal locking clip.

The car seat is anchored at the top by a tether strap, which should be bolted to the car frame. The seats are equipped with a five-point harness or a shield. There are two types of shields. A T-Shield is a padded T-shaped or triangular shield attached to the shoulder straps. A Tray-Shield is a wide, rounded shield that looks like an armrest, which is attached to the car seat with arms, and swings down around the child. These shields must be low to restrain the child's hips. The shoulder-harness straps should be kept snug. If a plastic harness clip is provided, it should be pulled up to armpit level to keep the straps on the shoulders.

Young school-age children (over 4 to 5 years of age, over 40 lb/18 kg)

It's safest to keep your child in a car seat for as long as possible. However, when the child's head is more than halfway above the top of the car seat, the child has outgrown the seat. In this position the child may suffer a whiplash neck injury in a car crash. Regular lap and shoulder seatbelts will not lie properly over a child's small hips and shoulders. Instead, the belts tend to lie over the abdomen and face or neck, which may put the child at risk of an injury from the seatbelt itself. To correct this, children should be placed in booster seats that properly reposition the regular seatbelts. The lap belt should ride over the hips rather than the abdomen, and the shoulder belt should cross the shoulders and body rather than the face or neck. If your car has combination lap and shoulder belts in the rear seats, choose a booster seat that allows for their use. If the rear seat has lap belts only, and no shoulder belts, use a booster seat with a shield; the lap belt wraps around the shield. Consider purchasing a booster with a large shield capable of cushioning the upper body and head as well as the lower body. Other devices are also commercially available to reposition the seatbelt.

Older school-age children

When the child's head is no longer protected by the back of the vehicle seat or head rest, he or she has outgrown the booster. Place the child in the regular lap and/or shoulder belt. Check that the child can touch nose to knees; this ensures that his or her spine can move with flexibility in case of a crash. The lap belt should lie low across the hips, well below the stomach. The shoulder belt should lie flat across the shoulders, not against the face or neck. If your child is still too small to fit properly in the adult seatbelt, devices are available to reposition the belt.

How can I protect my child as a pedestrian?

Pedestrian injuries are the leading cause of death in children four to eight years of age. Because the force of the impact is so great, severe multiple injuries are common, including head injuries. Children may be struck by cars when they dart out into traffic, especially where parked cars make it difficult for drivers to see them. Preventing pedestrian injury requires separating children from cars, slowing traffic in areas where children tend to cross the street, providing adult supervision for children unable to make safe decisions about street crossing, and training older children in street-crossing strategies.

Children younger than seven should cross streets only with adult supervision. Those seven to nine should not cross major streets, and should be taught to wait if there is approaching traffic. Older children should be taught how to watch for oncoming traffic, and not to dart out from between parked cars.

What about bicycle safety?

Bicycling is popular among both school-age children and adolescents; some surveys suggest that up to 80 percent of children own a bicycle. Death and disability from bicycle crashes are mostly due to head injury, when children either fall off their bikes or collide with fixed objects or motor vehicles. These are usually high-impact collisions. Two strategies are necessary to protect children from serious bicycle injuries: all bicyclists should wear helmets, and all bicyclists should receive training. Most children should not ride bicycles after dark; older children riding with their parents should have front and rear lights and reflective clothing when driving after dark, as should their parents.

Do helmets really offer much protection?

Studies suggest that a helmet may reduce the risk of head injury by 85 percent. In countries where cyclists must wear helmets by law, bicycle-related head injuries have decreased by more than 50 percent.

Bicycle helmets are specially designed to withstand high-impact collisions. Other types of helmets, such as football helmets, do not provide enough protection. Helmets should be approved by the American National Standards Institute (ANSI) or the Snell Memorial Foundation (Snell). Look for the logo on the inside of the helmet. Helmets should cover the top of the forehead, sitting not too far forward or too far backward. The straps should be snug without pinching. A helmet should not be used after it has been involved in a crash; even if it looks undamaged, it may have lost much of its strength.

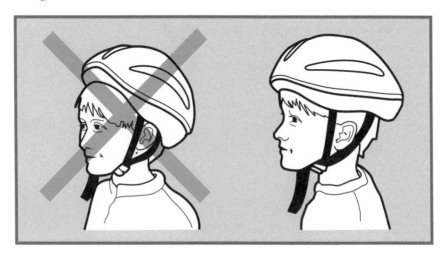

At what age should I buy my child a bicycle?

Consider allowing your child to ride a two-wheeled bike at about five or six years of age. Be sure the bike is the right size, using the following guidelines: sitting on the seat with both hands on the handlebars, your child must be able to place the balls of both feet on the ground; straddling the center bar, your child should be able to keep both feet flat on the ground with about an inch of clearance between crotch and bar; and the child should be able to grasp the hand brakes and apply enough pressure to stop the bike.

Under age eight, children should ride only with adult supervision, and off the street. Older children may ride on the street at their parents' discretion. Bicycling safely involves the following: riding with the traffic; riding single-file in a straight line, without swerving or moving between parked cars; stopping at all intersections; using hand signals when stopping and turning; checking over the shoulder when turning. Remember that your child is unlikely to obey safety rules if you yourself disregard them.

Injuries at Home

Most fatal and nonfatal injuries in children under age fifteen, especially preschool-age children, happen at home. The most common forms of home-injury deaths are suffocation, fires and burns, and drowning, while falls are the leading cause of non-fatal home injuries. Home-injury prevention programs have been found to be effective in increasing awareness and changing behavior, and decreasing home injuries.

How can I prevent injuries in the kitchen?

Whenever possible, keep toddlers out of the kitchen—especially during meal preparation, when hazards are greater and you may be too preoccupied to supervise closely. If necessary, provide a safe zone, for example a playpen. In addition,

- place an appliance latch on the refrigerator;

- avoid small refrigerator magnets, which can be a choking hazard;

- don't place an infant or older child on the counter;

- don't place an infant in an infant seat on a counter or other elevated area;

- keep garbage secured behind a latched door;

- rearrange storage areas so that dangerous equipment, cleaning compounds, and foods are kept in upper cabinets and drawers, and safe items in lower cabinets and drawers;

- install child-guard latches on drawers and cabinets that contain dangerous items;

- set aside one cabinet for safe items that the child can explore;

- keep knives away from counter edges;

- clean up spills immediately to avoid slipping.

How can I prevent burns?

If a playpen is located in the kitchen, keep it well away from the stove. As well,

- don't carry hot liquid when you're carrying a child;

- don't place hot items at the edge of the counter or table;

- use back burners of the stove when possible;

- turn pot handles inward on the stove;

- use stove-knob covers as a barrier to burner controls;

- keep your child away from ovens or other appliances that may be hot on the outside;

- never leave an appliance cord plugged into an outlet when the cord is disconnected from the appliance;

- keep appliances and electrical cords out of reach and away from the edges of counters;

- avoid heating formula or food in a microwave, as it may heat unevenly and scald a child's mouth;

- if you must use a microwave, set it to a low heat or for a brief time, mix the food thoroughly after heating, and test it before serving.

Do I have to do anything in the living room or family room?

Although these rooms may look safe, when children begin roughhousing or exploring they can easily hurt themselves. Therefore,

Preventing the tragedy of fire

How often have you heard about children dying in a house fire because there was no smoke alarm, or because the alarm's battery had been removed or had gone dead? Many people mean to install alarms but "don't get around to it." If you don't already have enough alarms, this should be high on your list of injury prevention.

If you're not sure how many alarms you need, check the alarm instructions, or consult your fire department. Alarms should be checked once a month, and it's wise to change the batteries once a year—pick a day and make it a ritual. (Let older children help, to reinforce their awareness of fire safety.)

Install a fire extinguisher in the kitchen, and in any other area where fire is particularly likely (such as the garage or workshop). Check it regularly, to be sure it's still charged. Everyone old enough to handle the extinguishers should know how to remove them from their mountings and use them.

Get pamphlets on fire safety from your local fire department or first-aid agency, and teach your children what to do in a fire. Practise fire drill as a game. If any parts of your home have limited access (such as upper bedrooms with a single staircase), consult your fire department about emergency escape equipment.

Even if you never have a fire, the safety you practise at home will set a valuable example for your children.

- make sure all furniture is stable;

- check that handles and knobs are secure, and large enough that they don't present a choking hazard;

- cover sharp edges of furniture, for example, coffee tables, with corner guards;

- avoid glass-topped tables;

- install wall-to-wall carpeting, or ensure that the rug has a non-skid backing;

- keep ashtrays, matches, and cigarettes out of reach;

- keep heavy objects such as bookends out of reach;

- keep audio and visual equipment like VCRs, CD players, and televisions out of reach;

- install a VCR guard on the cassette loader to keep prying fingers out;

- keep window-blind and drapery cords out of reach so children can't strangle;

- avoid falls from windows by installing window guards or locking devices that won't allow a window opening of more than 4 inches (10 cm).

What should I do about electrical cords and appliances?

Use as few electrical cords as possible, and move them behind furniture so they can't be chewed or tugged. Avoid using extension cords. As well,

- cover electrical outlets with shields, and place heavy furniture in front of them;

- don't leave a lamp without a bulb;

- keep hot lightbulbs out of your child's reach;

- install protective barriers on fireplaces, heaters, stoves, and radiators;

- avoid using space heaters; if you must use one, be sure it turns off automatically if toppled, and turn it off when adults are out of the room or asleep; keep all heaters out of reach of children.

Are playpens and baby walkers safe?

A playpen may be used as a safe area, but be sure it has fine mesh sides with openings of less than ¼ inch (½ cm), or vertical slats less than 2⅜ inches (6 cm) apart. The playpen should always be fully open so that it can't collapse and so that there's no space between the mattress and the mesh side.

Ideally, you should avoid using a baby walker. If you must use one, block off stairways and outer doorways; don't use it on uneven floors, carpets, or thresholds; and clear objects off tables. Keep any child in a walker away from ovens, space heaters, and fireplaces; keep hot liquids away from children in walkers. Never leave a child in a walker unattended.

What about the dining room?

Follow the same precautions as in the living room. In addition,

- keep heavy or fragile objects out of reach;

- don't use long tablecloths that overhang the table;

- be sure the highchair has a wide base so it won't easily topple over;

- keep the child strapped in when he or she is in the highchair;

- never leave the child unattended in the highchair.

And the bedroom?

Take the same measures as in the living room. As well,

- don't use infant cushions;

- never let infants sleep on an adult bed, because they can become trapped between the bed and wall and suffocate;

- don't leave an infant on a waterbed;

- don't leave an infant unattended on a changing table;

- use covered wastebaskets, or don't place hazardous items in an open wastebasket (for example, plastic bags, small or sharp items, rubber bands, batteries, balloons);

- avoid toy chests, or install a spring-loaded device to hold the lid open at any angle, so that it won't automatically snap shut; drill air holes in the body of the box;

- better yet, use open bins, baskets, and shelves for toy storage;

- don't put heavy items in a child's bedroom;

- keep window-blind or drapery cords out of reach by clipping them to themselves or to the blinds with clamping devices, wrapping them around cleats near the top of the blinds, tying the cords to themselves, or installing tie-down devices on the windowsills;

- don't place a crib, playpen, chair, or bed within reach of a window-blind or drapery cord;

- install grilles or child-resistant screens on windows.

How can I be sure my child's bed is safe?

Cribs should meet the standards of the Consumer Product Safety Commission. Slats should be no more than 2⅜ inches (6 cm) apart, wood surfaces should be free of splinters and cracks and have lead-free paint, and end panels should be of a material that won't splinter. There should be no corner posts, as these can catch clothing; no crossbars on the sides; and no decorative cutouts that might trap a child. The sides should be hand-operated with a locking latch that can't be released accidentally. The minimum rail height should be 22 inches (56 cm) from the top of the rail to the mattress set at the lowest level, and when the sides are lowered they should still be 4 inches (10 cm) above the mattress. The mattress should be the same size as the crib, so there are no gaps to catch an arm or leg.

When using the crib,

- never leave the rails down when the baby is in the crib;

- use bumper pads around the entire crib until the baby begins to stand, and then remove them;

- begin to lower the crib mattress before the baby can sit unassisted; have it at its lowest point before the baby can stand;

- don't hang any crib toys within reach;

- remove any crib toys strung across the crib when the child is beginning to push up on hands and knees, or is five months of age;

- don't leave large toys in the crib, as the baby may use them as steps to climb out;

- place a rug or carpet under the crib;

- use netting or safe extenders on the top of the crib if the baby has tried to climb out;

- remove the child from the crib when he or she is 35 inches (90 cm) tall.

A toddler's bed should have safety rails, and should be placed at least two feet (half a meter) from windows, heating vents, radiators, wall lamps, drapery, and window-blind cords.

Bunk beds should have guard rails next to the wall and at both ends on the upper and lower bunks, and on the outer side on the upper bunk. Guardrails should extend at least 5 inches (13 cm) above the mattress, and the mattresses should sit on cross supports of wood slats, metal straps, or sturdy wires. Attach additional boards to the bunk bed to close up any space more than 3½ inches (9 cm) wide between the lower edge of the guard rails and the upper edge of the bed frame, to prevent entrapment. Children under six should not sleep in the top bunk, and rough play should not be allowed on either bunk.

 ## What about safety in the bathroom?

It's a good idea to keep children out of the bathroom when they're not using it, by keeping the door closed and installing a hook-and-eye latch or doorknob cover on the outside. Don't have any inside locks that you can't open from the outside. In addition,

- keep the toilet lid closed with a safety latch;

- use non-slip bathmats;

- use a covered wastebasket;

- keep medications and cleaning products in a latched cabinet, and keep any other harmful items out of reach;

- keep the phone number of a poison control center handy; have syrup of ipecac on hand (to induce vomiting) in case the poison control center advises you to administer it.

 Are there special precautions for the bathtub?
Never leave an infant or child unattended in the water, even in a special tub or seat, until the child is at least five years old. If you're bathing an infant or child, ignore all other interruptions; don't leave "for a moment" to answer the door or telephone. Never leave water in the tub when it's not in use. As well,

- use an infant tub for younger infants, and a supporting ring for older ones;

- be sure the tub bottom is slip-proof, or add non-slip decals;

- set your household water heater no higher than 120°F (50°C);

- use an anti-scald device to keep the water temperature below 120°F (50°C);

- turn on the cold tap before the hot one, and turn off the hot tap before the cold one;

- use a single tap rather than separate hot and cold ones, if possible;

- install a protective cover over the tub spout to prevent bumps and burns;

- test the water temperature before placing the child in the bath;

- don't leave soap and shampoo on the edge of the tub.

- keep electrical appliances away from children;

- keep electrical appliances away from water, and don't leave them plugged in;

- install ground-fault circuit interrupters to cut power instantly in case of an electrical problem.

Do I need to do anything in hallways and on stairs?

Stairs are very dangerous to young children, and often very appealing. You should put gates at the top and bottom of the stairs when your infant begins to crawl; gates at the top should be permanently installed, but those at the bottom may be portable. Gates should have vertical slats no more than 2⅜ inches (6 cm) apart, or be made of fine mesh or plexiglass. If the gate has diamond-shaped openings, they should be no more than 1½ inches (4 cm) wide. Avoid accordion-style gates with large diamond-shaped openings, as they may trap a child's fingers.

With older children, keep stairs clear of objects and be sure both stairs and hallways are well lit at night. Install carpet with non-skid backing in the halls, on the stairs, and at the foot of each staircase. In addition,

- keep plants out of reach;

- be sure railings are secure, and check that upright posts are no more than 4 inches (10 cm) apart;

- keep hallways clear of clutter, and floors in good repair;

- don't overwax floors;

- clean up spills immediately to avoid slipping.

What about other parts of the house?

The following areas should be off limits: garage, basement, greenhouse, workshop, exercise room, laundry room. In the laundry room, keep the dryer door closed at all times, and keep detergents, bleach, and other products in a cabinet out of reach. Keep children away from standing water in buckets, diaper pails, and other containers. In general,

- never leave children home alone;

- keep doors locked at all times, whether you're at home or away;

- keep all doors, sliders, and screens secured with toddler-proof locks, and mark glass doors with decals;

- don't keep guns in your home; if you must keep one, have it locked up, inaccessible, and unloaded, and store the bullets in a separate location.

Water Safety

Drowning is a major cause of death in children. Drowning rates are highest for children under five and for adolescents over fifteen. About half of all drownings occur in lakes, ponds, rivers, and oceans, and half in residential swimming pools. Young children don't understand the dangers of falling into water, and may not be able to call for help. Most young victims drown during short periods of time (often less than five minutes) when no adult is supervising. While precautions can help make children safe around water, nothing can replace adult supervision at all times. In case something does happen, you and anyone else who cares for your child should learn basic water-rescue techniques and cardiopulmonary resuscitation (CPR). Any child who may have aspirated (inhaled) water should have immediate medical attention; even if the child seems fine, the water may have caused lung damage.

How can I make my swimming pool safe?

It's estimated that effective barriers around swimming pools would prevent up to 70 percent of pool drownings. Fences should be at least 5 feet (1.5 meters) high, with openings no greater than 4 inches (10 cm) wide. Gates should be self-closing and self-latching, with latches placed high enough that small children can't reach them. Fences enclosing the pool, separating it from the rest of the yard and the house, are more effective than fences enclosing the entire property, but be sure the fence doesn't block your view of the pool.

Does drownproofing work?

"Drownproofing" children under four years of age is controversial, and has not been proven to ensure adequate swimming skills or to make children safer in the water. In chilly waters the physical exertion of "drownproofing" techniques is likely to lead to hypothermia (loss of body heat). On the other hand, swimming lessons for preschoolers may promote a false sense of security for both parent and child. Therefore, swimming lessons are not recommended until children are four or five years of age. Even in older children, it's not known whether formal swimming lessons decrease the risk of drowning.

Boating injuries are more common among young adults and adults than children. The two most effective precautions are using personal flotation devices (PFDs) of the right size, and not operating a boat under the influence of alcohol. Up to 50 percent of boating fatalities involve alcohol. Note that drinking on a small boat (without living accommodation) is just as illegal as drinking in a car, even when the boat is moored.

Playground Injuries

Most playground injuries are minor, but up to one-quarter may be severe, involving head injuries and broken bones. Most playground injuries are caused by falls from playground equipment (especially climbing equipment) to the surface. Concrete and asphalt surfaces are more dangerous than sand and similar artificial surfaces. Equipment should be inspected for projecting bolts and sharp edges, as well as overall maintenance. Equipment should be placed so that collisions are unlikely. Currently, guidelines for the installation and maintenance of playgrounds are voluntary; you may wish to evaluate the safety of your local public and school playgrounds for yourself.

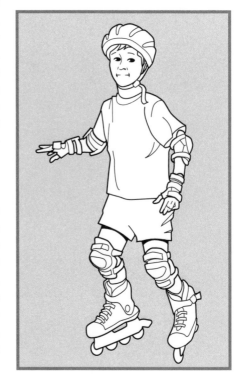

How dangerous is in-line skating?

Most childhood in-line skating injuries occur in children ten to fourteen years of age, on roads and sidewalks. Almost half of these result in broken bones or dislocations, while the remainder consist of lesser injuries such as sprains, cuts, bruises, and scrapes. The child's hand or arm is most often injured. Children should wear a helmet, knee pads, elbow pads, and wrist pads. They should only skate in traffic-free areas such as rinks, parks, and playgrounds.

Plan for the best, prepare for the worst

No matter what precautions you take, you should still be prepared to deal with injuries. Keep a first-aid kit at home and in your car, and anywhere else you're likely to need one (note that small "fanny-pack" kits are available). Take a first-aid course that includes CPR, and encourage babysitters and others who care for your child to do the same. For more information on first-aid courses, and specific advice for life-threatening emergencies, see Chapter 18, "Emergency First Aid."

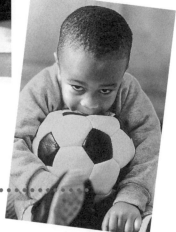

CHAPTER 14

Diseases and Medical Conditions

• •

Afull listing of the diseases and conditions that may affect children is beyond the scope of this book, but the following are problems frequently encountered, or of particular concern. They are presented alphabetically for ease of reference.

Topics covered are:

- asthma;
- bronchiolitis;
- chicken pox (varicella);
- colds (viral upper-respiratory infections);
- croup;
- diphtheria;
- fifth disease (erythema infectiosum);
- haemophilus influenzae B (epiglottitis);

- hepatitis;
- measles;
- mumps;
- pertussis (whooping cough);
- pneumonia;
- roseola;
- rubella (German measles);
- scarlet fever and strep throat;
- tetanus.

Asthma
• • • • • • • • • • • •
Approximately 5 to 10 percent of children have at least mild asthma at some period in their lives. It's a leading cause of chronic illness in childhood, the most common reason for admission to a children's hospital, and a major cause of school absenteeism. Fortunately, many children outgrow it.

Asthma is characterized by recurrent bouts of wheezing, coughing, and shortness of breath. The airways are "hyperactive"—they react more than normal to various stimuli, and respond with narrowing and inflammation. The stimuli include such things as smoke, dust and paint, exercise, colds, and even cold air. The most common offending agent in young children is a cold. Secondhand smoke is another common trigger, especially in infants. Older children are more likely to be allergic, reacting to pets, pollens, and molds; humidifiers are a source of molds and must be cleaned regularly. The season of the year is significant: early spring suggests tree allergies as a trigger, late spring suggests grasses, and mid-August to the first frost suggests ragweed. Emotional factors are rarely important in causing childhood asthma.

When and how does asthma first appear?

The vast majority of asthmatic children develop symptoms by age five. The typical case is a young child who develops a cold, and several days later begins to cough, wheeze, and breathe quickly. You may hear a wheeze when the child breathes out. The child may be short of breath, with the lower ribs sucking in on each breath. Another common example is the child who wheezes and coughs with exercise, especially in a cold environment such as a hockey rink. Some children never wheeze but develop a cough, usually dry and nonproductive, when exposed to triggers. These are the children who have a history of a "cold" that always goes to the chest. Frequently one parent has a similar history, and there may also be a family history of recurrent bronchitis.

How is asthma treated?

Most asthma is mild and can be controlled by medication. The aims are to dilate the narrowed airways and decrease their inflammation. "Bronchodilators" (airway openers) such as salbutamol may be inhaled from a metered-dose inhaler or a nebulizer (a small machine that uses air to force medication into the child's lungs). They may also be taken orally; this is less effective, but convenient for infants with mild wheezing. Bronchodilators are usually given after wheezing starts, but if they are taken before exercise they may prevent wheezing.

Anti-inflammatory drugs such as cromoglycate or inhaled steroids are given by inhalation, but must be taken regularly to be effective. They are intended to prevent asthma attacks. After inhaling steroids, the mouth should be rinsed. Oral or intravenous steroids may be helpful during an acute attack, but they have to be used with caution.

Aggressive treatment is the key to controlling asthma. It's extremely important that you understand the triggers to your child's disease, and follow medication instructions carefully.

Do allergy shots help prevent asthma?

Allergy shots should be considered only for clear-cut pollen-related asthma that hasn't improved after four to six months of inhaled anti-inflammatories. Most children with specific pollen allergies do respond to anti-inflammatories and don't require allergy shots.

Bronchiolitis

Bronchiolitis is a common disease of infancy and is responsible for many admissions to hospital. It occurs in children under two years of age, and usually under six months old. Respiratory syncytial virus is the most common cause, but most infants with respiratory syncytial virus will not develop bronchiolitis. Most cases occur in winter and spring. Usually the child has a mild cold for a few days, and then develops more coughing and has trouble breathing; as he or she breathes out, a wheeze or whistle may be heard. The child breathes more quickly than normal, and the lower ribs are pulled inwards with each breath. There may also be a fever.

Does a child with bronchiolitis have to go to hospital?

If the child isn't too distressed, home therapy with a humidifier may be enough. He or she may be given an oral bronchodilator to open the airway. (This is more likely to help if there's a family history of asthma.) More distressed infants are admitted to hospital and may receive intravenous fluids as well as moisturized air or oxygen. It may be necessary to administer medication through an inhalation mask to widen the airways and ease the child's breathing. Antibiotics are of no value in a routine case of bronchiolitis. A chest X ray may be done to be sure there's no secondary infection such as pneumonia. Bronchiolitis takes seven to ten days to resolve, but a small percentage of children have recurrent episodes; this suggests the child is asthmatic, especially if there's a family history of asthma.

Chicken Pox

Chicken pox (varicella) is a very contagious viral infection; more than 90 percent of the population has been infected with it. It occurs most frequently in late winter or early spring.

The infection is spread by close contact with an infected person. The illness usually appears fourteen to sixteen days after exposure, but the interval may be as short as ten days or as long as twenty-one days. Chicken pox is infectious starting twenty-four hours before the rash appears, and until the spots have crusted over (generally five to seven days).

In children, chicken pox usually begins with a low fever, followed by the appearance of a rash. The rash starts off as small, raised red bumps that later become little fluid-filled blisters. The blisters then form dry brown crusts, which fall off. Repeated groups of these sores form over the next few days. The rash most often starts on the trunk and face and spreads to the rest of the body. It may affect the mouth, eyelids, and genital area. Chicken pox is very itchy, but the illness is usually mild in children. The diagnosis is usually obvious from the rash. Blood tests are very rarely needed.

Can chicken pox lead to more serious problems?

The most common complication is bacterial infection of one or more spots. The area appears red, swollen, and painful, and antibiotic treatment may be needed. Other complications (such as pneumonia and encephalitis) are rare, and happen mainly in adults, especially those with immune-system problems. The chicken pox virus stays in the body after the rash has cleared, but is not infectious to others. Occasionally it is reactivated and causes shingles (zoster), which usually looks like groups of little blisters in one area of the body. This condition is not serious but can be persistent and very painful.

Isn't chicken pox dangerous to an unborn child?

Chicken pox in the first twenty weeks of pregnancy may result in severe damage to the fetus, but that occurs in fewer than 3 percent of pregnancies complicated by chicken pox. In addition, if a woman gets chicken pox a few days before or after delivering a baby, the baby may become seriously ill, because he or she has not yet developed a strong immune system. Any pregnant woman who is exposed to chicken pox and has not had the illness before (or isn't sure she has) should seek medical attention as soon as possible.

Since chicken pox is a viral illness, antibiotics aren't useful unless the spots become infected. Antiviral medication is available but isn't usually prescribed for normal, healthy children. Antihistamines, calamine, or other lotions may help prevent itching and scratching. People of all ages who have decreased immunity, as well as adults and adolescents who are exposed to chicken pox, should contact their physicians as soon as possible, since preventive treatment may be indicated. A vaccine for chicken pox has recently become available in the United States.

What do I do if my child has chicken pox?

Current recommendations are to keep the child out of school or day care until all the spots have crusted over, or for six days after the rash begins (whichever comes first). However, many experts believe isolation isn't necessary, because the disease is most contagious before the rash appears, and because if people aren't infected during childhood they'll be at risk of more serious infection later on.

Colds

"Common colds," or upper-respiratory infections, are the most common acute infections in children. Infants and preschool children average six to ten episodes a year, while schoolchildren and adolescents average three to five. Children who attend daycare or live in crowded homes get even more colds. Since colds are spread by large droplets, often transferred from nose to hand, hand-washing is the most effective way to avoid spreading them.

Colds aren't serious in themselves, but can lead to complications such as ear infections and pneumonia. A fever at the beginning of a cold is normal, but a fever developing several days later suggests a secondary infection.

How can I treat a cold?

Since colds are caused by viruses, antibiotics are of no use in treating them. They are also of no value in preventing secondary bacterial infections. Bed rest is of no benefit if the child feels well enough to be up and active. Acetaminophen should be given for the fatigue, aches, and irritability that may accompany fever. Infants may have difficulty feeding if their noses are blocked, since they normally breathe through their noses. Small babies with stuffed-up noses may benefit from saline drops before feedings, but antihistamine–decongestant and other over-the-counter combinations have been shown to cause no significant improvement in children's symptoms. There is no truth to the notion that milk and dairy products increase the congestion or nasal secretions. Moreover, it's important that a child with a fever have plenty of fluids, to avoid dehydration. You may have to supply beverages often, in small amounts, if the child is reluctant to drink. Humidifiers may provide some relief from nasal stuffiness, but only a small amount of humidity is necessary as most of the moisture is deposited in the nose. Steam should be avoided because of the risk of burns.

Croup

Croup (acute laryngotracheobronchitis) is an acute but usually brief viral illness of the upper airway. It usually occurs between the ages of six months and three years, particularly around two years, and is most common in the late fall and winter. Typically the child has a mild cold for a few days, or awakens suddenly at night with a harsh barky cough and a hoarse voice. There is a low fever, and the child may make a harsh noise when breathing in. The child is frequently upset and crying. Cough medicine will not relieve the cough.

What can I do about croup?

For immediate relief, take the child into the washroom and turn on the shower so the room becomes full of moisture; you can sit there and read the child a story, which is reassuring and comforting. Another remedy is to take the child outside into the cool night air. The majority of croup is treated at home and does not require hospitalization.

A child who still has difficult breathing (not just noisy breathing) should be taken to the hospital. Treatment there may consist of an inhalation or mask of medication to decrease the airway inflammation and relieve the breathing problem. Humidified air or oxygen may also be given. Recently, the traditional "croup tents" have been replaced by other ways of supplying humidified air. Another method of decreasing inflammation is to give an injection of dexamethasone.

Diphtheria

Diphtheria is an acute bacterial infection that may result only in symptoms similar to those of the common cold, or may totally obstruct the upper airway, resulting in suffocation. The bacteria produce a poisonous compound (toxin) that can attack the heart muscle, cause paralysis, or even lead to kidney failure. Fortunately, immunization has made this disease extremely rare in North America.

Symptoms include fever, rapid pulse, swollen neck glands, and sometimes a thick yellow discharge from the nose, but the most distinctive indication is a grayish membrane on the throat and tonsils. Treatment requires hospitalization.

Epiglottitis, see Haemophilus Influenzae B

Erythema Infectiosum, see Fifth Disease

Fifth Disease

Fifth disease (erythema infectiosum) is caused by a virus and most commonly affects school-age children, often in late winter or spring. It's spread by close contact, and symptoms begin to appear four to fourteen days later—usually mild fever and sore throat, followed by a rash. The rash on the face is bright red and mainly on the cheeks, giving a characteristic "slapped face" appearance. A lacy rash may be seen on the arms, legs, and trunk, and may come and go over a few weeks. The disease is most contagious before the rash appears. Joint pain is unusual in children but is quite common in women. The infection can also cause a rash without fever, or a mild coldlike illness with no rash.

Diagnosis is made by a physical examination, but may be difficult if the typical symptoms aren't present. Because it's generally such a mild illness, routine blood tests are not necessary.

Can fifth disease cause complications?

In normal, healthy children, complications are extremely rare, but children with immune deficiency or blood diseases such as sickle cell anemia are at risk of developing very severe anemia. If a woman is infected with the virus during the first half of pregnancy, the fetus may become very anemic, and may even die. Fewer than 10 percent of infected fetuses become anemic; the reason why only some babies are affected is not well understood. During the second half of pregnancy, the risk to the fetus is almost non-existent. The virus does not cause birth defects.

What do I do for a child with fifth disease?

There is no treatment for the disease, but children or fetuses with anemia may require blood transfusions. Children can attend school or day care, since they are no longer infectious once the rash appears. It's very difficult for pregnant women to avoid exposure, since the disease may be difficult to diagnose, and is infectious before the rash shows up. However, the overall risk to the pregnancy is low. Blood tests are available if a woman suspects she's been infected or exposed. If she has been infected, the pregnancy should be closely monitored.

Pregnant women, and children with immune or blood diseases, should seek medical attention if they may have been infected with or exposed to fifth disease.

German Measles, see Rubella

Haemophilus Influenzae B

Haemophilus influenzae B (epiglottitis) is an infection of the upper airway causing inflammation of the epiglottis, the flap that covers the upper airway when we swallow. It's due to a bacteria called Haemophilus influenzae B. The frequency of this disease has decreased significantly since the introduction of vaccination against this bacteria. The child, usually over three, awakens with difficulty breathing in, and appears ill and is frightened. Swallowing is also difficult, and as the disease progresses the child may drool as even saliva is hard to swallow. The child tends to sit upright and fights for every breath. In addition to the danger of a totally blocked airway, children with H. influenzae B may develop meningitis (brain inflammation). Although H. influenzae B is now a rare disease, thanks to immunization that is almost 100 percent effective, it's a medical emergency and the child must be rushed to hospital.

Hepatitis

Hepatitis is a liver infection caused by several viruses and showing up in several forms. Symptoms may (or may not) include jaundice (yellowing of the skin and eyes), weakness, loss of appetite, brownish urine, whitish stools, nausea, discomfort in the abdomen, and fever.

Hepatitis A is highly contagious, and is spread by contamination from blood or stool. The only treatment is bed rest. Most people recover fully, and have immunity thereafter.

Hepatitis B may be more serious. Some people ("carriers") have no symptoms at all, but can infect others. A few people develop "fulminant" (acute) hepatitis and can die of liver failure; others get a simmering chronic infection that can ultimately lead to cirrhosis of the liver or liver cancer.

 Who gets hepatitis B?
Hepatitis B is spread by body fluids, often through sexual contact or illicit drug

use. Newborns of infected mothers are at significant risk, as are some adolescents. Mild cases are treated with bed rest and a high-calorie diet, but severe cases may require complex treatment in hospital. The best treatment is prevention; immunization produces immunity in 95 percent of healthy children.

Lockjaw, see Tetanus

Measles

Measles is a viral infection that is preventable by immunization. In recent years, outbreaks have occurred among preschool children as well as high-school and college students.

Measles is spread by personal contact and shows up after eight to twelve days. The first symptoms are high fever, runny nose, cough, and red eyes. After three or four days, small, painless white spots appear in the mouth. A reddish rash starts on the scalp, hairline, and neck, and spreads downwards. After a few days, the rash fades and disappears, sometimes with fine peeling of the skin. Affected children usually look sick and are quite miserable. They are contagious from three to five days before the rash appears, until four days later.

Diagnosis can be made based on an examination of the child. Public-health authorities should be informed by the doctor so that they can try to prevent the disease's spread, since measles can be a severe illness.

Does measles lead to complications?

Complications are most likely to occur in younger children, and include ear infections, pneumonia, croup, and diarrhea. More serious complications are rare, although very occasionally encephalitis (brain inflammation) follows measles. Life-threatening complications are more common in children with immune problems.

What do I do if my child has measles?

No specific treatment has been shown to be effective for children who are not malnourished. (In developing countries, where malnutrition is a major problem, vitamin A injections are useful.) The child should not go to school or day care for four days after the rash starts (children usually feel too sick anyway). If a bacterial infection such as an ear infection or pneumonia develops, antibiotics should be prescribed. Immunization of people who

157

were in contact with the child may be recommended. People who think they have measles or may have been exposed to somebody with measles should contact their doctors as soon as possible.

Mumps

Mumps is a viral illness, preventable through immunization, that tends to occur in school-age children, especially in late winter and early spring. It's spread by coughing, sneezing, and talking, and shows up about two weeks after exposure. Many youngsters show no obvious sign of infection, but others develop swollen cheeks from infected saliva glands; there may also be headache, fever, diarrhea, and irritability. The mouth may feel dry, and eating and talking may hurt. The disease is infectious from about a day before symptoms appear until about three days after the swelling goes down.

Like many viral infections, the disease is more severe in older children and adults. Painfully inflamed testicles (orchitis) occur in about a quarter of boys past puberty. Luckily, sterility is rare, but loud complaint is not! In girls past puberty, the ovaries may be involved. Viral meningitis and encephalitis are relatively common following mumps, but they tend to be mild, with severe long-term consequences being rare.

 What can I do for a child with mumps?

There is no specific treatment, but soft foods and lots of fluids will help prevent mouth discomfort. Frequent toothbrushing and use of mouthwash may prevent gingivitis (gum inflammation). An icepack wrapped in a towel may relieve the soreness of the swollen glands.

Pertussis

Pertussis (whooping cough) is a highly contagious bacterial disease that begins like a normal cough but develops, after about fourteen days, into a series of repetitive coughs, as the air passages become clogged with mucus. The child may turn red, or even blue, before finally taking in a long breath, perhaps with a crowing noise; this is the "whoop" that gives the disease its popular name. Following the spasms, the child has watery eyes, and mucus streaming from the nose, and may vomit. The cough is worse at night, but running around during the day may precipitate a coughing spasm. This period lasts two weeks and is the most severe. It's then followed by a two-week interval of recovery.

Unfortunately, whenever the child has a cold over the following few months the cough may return, although for a shorter time. Frequently one of the adults in the house is a "reservoir" of this infection, which then spreads to the children.

How serious is pertussis?

The most severe cases are in younger infants, especially those under six months. The frequency and severity of pertussis have decreased since the introduction of vaccination. Antibiotics don't cure this disease; it must run its natural course. Untreated pertussis is contagious for three weeks from the start of the cough, but a course of erythromycin will eradicate the bacteria and shorten the infectious period. Most children should receive this drug to make them noncontagious, although it won't affect their illness. Other members of the family should also receive erythromycin, as there is evidence that if it's given before the onset of the disease, it may prevent it. Although older children and adults eventually recover, pertussis can persist for a long time; the Chinese call it "the hundred-day cough." If the cough begins in the fall, it frequently persists, on and off, until spring.

What can I do for a child with pertussis?

Don't give cough medications, as the coughing is necessary to clear the airway. If the coughing causes vomiting, try giving smaller, more frequent meals (but not right after a coughing bout). A coughing baby should lie face down with the foot of the crib raised; older children are usually more comfortable sitting up and leaning forward.

Can pertussis have serious complications?

Very occasionally, the disease leads to secondary pneumonia, seizures, or coma. In young infants the lack of oxygen during a coughing spell may rarely cause brain damage. A baby with a very severe cough may need hospitalization so that oxygen can be supplied. If a child is turning blue during coughing spells, get medical help at once.

Pneumonia

Pneumonia is an infection in the lungs. It may be caused by many bacteria and viruses, or may be due to chemicals, recurrent vomiting, or aspiration (breathing stomach contents into the lungs). Commonly the child has a mild

159

cold for a few days before the lung infection sets in. Symptoms include fever, rapid breathing, coughing, and increasing illness. As the disease progresses, the child may develop grunting breathing and the lower ribs may be sucked in during inhalation. The younger the child, the sicker and more distressed he or she is likely to be. A physician may be able to hear sounds in the child's chest that suggest pneumonia, but in a crying infant these are easily missed. A young infant who is ill, with difficult, rapid breathing and sucked-in ribs, may not be difficult to diagnose, but an older child with no more than a cough, low temperature, and mild illness may have a viral pneumonia that can be diagnosed only by a chest X ray. Even then, the X ray can't identify the type of pneumonia. Sometimes a second X ray is done after the end of therapy, to be sure the disease has resolved.

What treatment is there for pneumonia?

The majority of children (other than infants) do not need to be hospitalized; they improve rapidly and recover totally. Although most cases are viral, it's hard to distinguish viral pneumonia from bacterial pneumonia, so an antibiotic (usually amoxicillin) is given on the chance that it will help. A particular type of pneumonia due to an organism called "mycoplasma pneumonia" is common in older children, and especially teenagers; it responds to erythromycin. Cough suppressants have not been shown to be valuable in treating the cough that comes with pneumonia.

Does pneumonia tend to come back?

Recurrent pneumonia is uncommon in children, and when it occurs there may be some underlying cause. It's important to establish whether the child is generally well or seems to have a chronic disease. If the child is well, recurrent pneumonia may suggest asthma, especially if it's associated with wheezing. If the child isn't gaining weight, it may suggest cystic fibrosis. If the child is neurologically handicapped, it may suggest recurrent aspiration. If one area of the lung is affected repeatedly—and especially if the pneumonia is associated with some lung collapse—the possibility of a foreign body (such as a peanut) must be considered.

Roseola
············

Roseola is caused by a virus called "human herpes virus-6." It occurs most commonly in children aged six months to two years, and is rare in children over the age of four. Infections occur throughout the year. It's believed that children are usually infected by family members or caregivers who have the virus but aren't ill. The disease shows up about nine days after exposure. Children are probably infectious before the rash appears.

The child develops a very high fever, with no other symptoms until the fever goes down a few days later and a fine pink or reddish rash starts on the body and spreads to the neck, arms, and legs. It lasts hours to days. Occasionally there is some stomach upset or a runny nose. Often the child is irritable while the fever peaks but playful and lively at other times.

The diagnosis is made by examining and following the child. Frequently, the cause of the fever becomes obvious only when the rash appears. Blood tests are not necessary.

Are there complications to roseola?

The most common complication is seizures that may occur at the time of the fever (see Chapter 5, "Fever"). Roseola may occur more than once; the virus probably remains in the body and is then reactivated.

What can I do for a child with roseola?

No specific treatment is available. Any young child with a high fever (with or without seizures) should be seen by a physician, to ensure that no more serious illness is the cause. There is no need to isolate the child.

Rubella

Rubella (German measles) is a viral infection that most often occurs in late winter and early spring. It spreads directly from person to person and shows up fourteen to twenty-one days after exposure.

In children, rubella is usually a very mild disease. The rash, usually the first sign that the child is ill, appears on the face and hairline, and later spreads to the rest of the body. Initially it consists of fine, pale pink spots, which may join up as the rash spreads. It lasts about three days. The child may have a low fever and swollen lymph glands. Joint pain is unusual in children; it's not uncommon in adolescents and adults, especially females.

Rubella can be difficult to diagnose, especially since the rash is similar to those caused by many other viral infections. Blood tests are seldom necessary, except when a pregnant woman may have been exposed or infected.

Complications of rubella in the patient are extremely rare. However, if a pregnant woman becomes infected, the baby may be severely affected by problems such as diminished birth weight, mental retardation, deafness, cataracts, heart defects, damaged retinas, and later complications such as diabetes mellitus and thyroid disease. In order to prevent exposure during pregnancy, immunization of children is essential. Any pregnant woman who thinks she has been exposed to or infected with rubella should seek medical attention as soon as possible.

What can I do for a child with rubella?

No treatment is available for rubella. Children should be kept away from school or day care for seven days after the rash starts.

Scarlet Fever
....

Scarlet fever is a bacterial infection. It's the same illness as strep throat, but with a skin rash. It's most common in school-age children, but can affect any age group. Both scarlet fever and strep throat occur throughout the year but are more frequent in the late fall, winter, and early spring. They are spread by infected individuals, and symptoms usually appear two to five days after exposure.

Symptoms include fever, headache, vomiting, and sore throat, and the child usually feels unwell. The mouth appears very red, and the tongue is initially covered with a thick white layer. After a couple of days, the tongue looks red and swollen ("strawberry tongue"). The lymph glands in the neck may be swollen and painful. In scarlet fever, a fine pink or red rash that feels like sandpaper appears in the first twelve to forty-eight hours and then spreads all over the body. The rash fades within four or five days, and the skin often peels, especially on the hands and feet.

If you think your child has scarlet fever or strep throat, consult your doctor. The diagnosis can be made by examining the child. A throat culture is useful to confirm a strep infection.

Are there complications to scarlet fever or strep throat?

Complications include ear infections, sinusitis, and pneumonia. A serious but rare complication is rheumatic fever, a disease that may occur a few weeks after the infection and can result in permanent heart damage. Antibiotic treatment of strep infections prevents this complication. Penicillin is highly effective, but other antibiotics are available for children who are allergic to penicillin. Although the child often feels much better within a couple of days, it is very important to complete the full course of antibiotics to prevent rheumatic fever. About 15 percent of children relapse and need a second course of antibiotics.

The child is no longer infectious after being treated with antibiotics for twenty-four hours. He or she can then go back to daycare or school, if well enough.

Strep Throat, see Scarlet Fever

Tetanus

Tetanus (lockjaw) is caused by a potent toxin produced by bacteria. It's usually contracted in a deep wound or puncture (such wounds are often not cleaned thoroughly). The risk is greater if the wound is from something dirty, such as a nail in a garden or farmyard.

The toxin attacks the nerves in the spinal cord, producing pain and muscle spasm at the site of the wound or more generally. It can tighten the facial muscles into a fixed grin—hence its popular name. There may be fever, paralysis, and asphyxiation. The disease is often fatal.

Immunization is very effective in providing long-lasting protection. Booster shots are required throughout life. Be sure your family's shots are up to date, and carry a record of the shots with you; if someone has a wound away from home, the attending doctor will want to be sure the patient's immunization is current. If a child has a deep or unclean wound, seek medical help at once.

Upper-Respiratory Infections, see Colds

Varicella, see Chicken Pox

Whooping Cough, see Pertussis

CHAPTER 15

Behavioral and Learning Problems

$\textbf{A}$ ll children display a wide variety of behaviors that concern or upset their parents at some time or other. One study showed that 8 percent of preschool children in England were judged to have a "behavior problem" by health professionals and parents. Another study in middle-class American families showed that 18 percent of children up to five years of age were diagnosed as having behavioral disturbances severe enough to warrant intervention. These included problems such as bedtime resistance, food refusal, resistance to toilet training, temper tantrums, aggression, shyness, hyperactivity, and undesirable habits such as thumb sucking. Individual behavioral symptoms are very common in young children, but whether they are labeled "problems" depends on the type, frequency, duration, and severity of the behavior. The full range of childhood behavioral problems is beyond the scope of this book; our focus will be on problems such as shyness, aggressiveness, conduct and oppositional-defiant disorders, and attention-deficit disorder, as well as learning disabilities, which are often associated with some of these disorders.

Shyness and Aggressiveness

The way a child reacts to unfamiliar situations is strongly affected by his or her inborn temperament or personality. After the age of two, when children start to interact with other children, it becomes easier to see a trend towards shyness or aggressiveness. Neither should be considered a problem unless it clearly and repeatedly interferes in the child's life and prevents effective problem solving. It's unlikely that any major problem will result from a child's inherent shyness or aggression before the age of six years. With preschoolers one can intervene by giving a shy child a small push, or gently restraining an aggressive child.

After the age of six, a child's shyness or aggressiveness can be more of a problem. Conduct and oppositional-defiant disorders are two forms of disruptive behavior that appear in middle childhood and adolescence. At this age antisocial behavior may be accompanied by some of the features of attention-deficit disorder with hyperactivity—including overactivity, short attention span, and lack of concentration. You can't expect to change your child's fundamental predisposition to shyness or aggressiveness, but you may be able to change the way he or she handles difficult situations.

How do I know if my child is shy?

Shy children often avoid others, and are usually timid, easily frightened, bashful, reserved, and hesitant to commit themselves. In social situations they are often silent, speak softly, and don't take the initiative. A shy child under the age of six may regularly be bossed about by other children, or may cling to parents, fail to make eye contact, or refuse to come downstairs when company visits. However, periods of shyness are normal at five or six months of age and again at two years. If any of the following symptoms lasts more than two months, the child may be exceedingly shy:

- repeated refusal to participate with peers;

- repeated incidents of being victimized by other children;

- preference for being left alone;

- excessive clinging to parents;

- persistent fearfulness or depression.

The shyness should be considered a problem if the symptoms persist.

What makes some children shy?

Many children appear to be shy almost from birth, and this "constitutional" shyness may continue for the rest of their lives. Others feel shy about physical differences, and may avoid situations in which they are made to feel uncomfortable.

Shy parents often produce shy children; in other words, a tendency to shyness may be inherited. Shyness may also develop in children who are overprotected by their parents or, conversely, overly criticized by them.

Children who are frequently threatened with punishment may react with fear and timidity. Those who are often teased by parents or siblings may become shy and shun social contact to avoid ridicule.

Low self-esteem can also be a factor. Children who feel insecure lack self-confidence. They are preoccupied with feeling safe and not getting hurt, and therefore don't develop social skills.

 What can I do to overcome my child's shyness?

You can start by setting an example of outgoing behavior. Let your child see you standing up for your rights when necessary, taking social risks, or seizing the initiative in difficult situations. A child who sees you starting conversations, making eye contact, and touching and staying close to people has an example to follow. Tell your child how you have overcome your shyness in various situations. For example, discuss how you introduce yourself to a stranger at a party or how you call the TV cable company to complain about being overcharged.

Be careful to tackle the child's various behaviors individually. Focus attention on each situation as it happens, not on the child's overall personality. *Do not* label your child shy. Talk about the situation, without blaming the child.

Reinforce any outgoing behavior you see in your child. Praise his or her efforts at being more independent and assertive. Point out how much you admire acts of self-confidence. For example, when your child says hello to a friend, encourage the behavior by saying, "You spoke to Mr. Smith very nicely. I liked the way you said, 'It was nice to meet you.'" Have the child's teacher help as well, rewarding behavior such as answering questions or raising a hand to volunteer information.

Rehearsing situations that your child finds stressful is helpful. For example, go over every step of meeting a new person, including the introduction and appropriate things to say. Teach your child words and techniques for joining other children's play: "Can I help you do that?" "I want to play too. Which team should I join?"

As well, help your child practice ways of coping with rejection. For example, when he or she is rejected by a social clique, explain that children who know each other often stick together and don't accept newcomers easily. "It doesn't mean that they don't like you, or that you're bad." Remind the child of successes in previous interactions.

Many shy children feel overwhelmed in large groups, so try to provide one-on-one or small-group activities. Pair shy children with younger playmates, who are less threatening. Organize special activities in which each child takes a turn, or provide large objects that require cooperation, such as see-saws.

If you realize your child is likely to be shy in a certain situation, try subtly to make it less threatening. Arrange an entrance into the event at a good time, and let the child acclimatize before you leave. Try to smooth the path but avoid either forcing or coddling. Pushing a child into a situation doesn't teach the child how to be outgoing, and a child who is ridiculed or ignored will feel rejected.

The Aggressive Child

Aggression can be defined as behavior that results in personal injury—psychological or physical—to someone else. For example, an aggressive child under the age of six may boss, tease, or hit other children and make them cry, or disturb everyone at a family gathering by demanding constant attention. Aggression is often triggered when a child wants something that another child has. Some preschool children even attack their parents over conflicts about feeding, bedtime, or the denial of something the child wants. There may be frequent temper tantrums. The child tends to be impulsive, immature, action-oriented, and inarticulate about feelings. Overaggressiveness is present in about 1 percent of ten-year-olds. Significantly aggressive behavior is classed as a conduct disorder (see below).

What makes a child aggressive?

Some experts believe that aggression is an inborn temperament, while others feel that young children learn aggressive habits by following examples set by parents, siblings, and peers. Faulty child-rearing practices, such as a combination of lax discipline and hostile attitudes in parents, can produce aggressive and poorly controlled children. Competition, exposure to TV violence, marital strife, and fathers absent from home for extended periods are other factors believed to foster aggression.

What can I do about an aggressive child?

The most direct way to encourage your child to get along with others is to praise him or her for doing so. Use a reward system, such as a star chart or tokens that can be traded in later for actual rewards. While rewarding good behavior and self-control, ignore aggressive acts that don't pose a threat to the physical safety of others; by paying attention to fighting or teasing, you may inadvertently reinforce this behavior. While ignoring the aggression, do give a great deal of attention to the *injured* party, showing your concern and empathy.

When you have to correct your child's aggression, direct your remarks at the situation, not the child in general. Children become angry and resentful if they feel they're being attacked.

Remember that children are influenced by the respect you display for the rights and feelings of others. If, for example, their parents argue and belittle each other, the children will likely relate in a similar manner.

How can I prevent aggressive episodes?

Teach your child that other people's rights and needs must be respected. A good time to do this is shortly after the child has ignored or violated someone else's rights; apart from direct discussion, one approach is through role-playing. Also, teach your child to "talk it out" rather than "fight it out." Give the child a list of things to do besides hitting when he or she feels upset, such as saying, "I'm not playing any more" and leaving the group.

Aggressive children often act before they think, so if you know your child tends to be aggressive in certain situations, take a few moments to discuss how you would like things to go. Teach the child to use aggression-inhibiting sentences when angry, such as "Count to ten" or "Talk, don't hit."

When your child abuses another child's rights, step in and correct the situation. Point out what's fair, gain everyone's commitment to fair play, and then withdraw. Try not to be punitive, but do get involved when a situation seems to be getting out of hand.

How should I punish aggression?

With younger children, a very effective form of punishment is "time out," in which the child is isolated—sent to his or her room, or sat on a chair—for a

---

Can television make children more aggressive?

Many studies have shown that television has an influence on the put-downs and aggressive behavior children use with each other. One study showed that heavy viewers of TV, especially action adventures and cartoons, were more aggressive and less cooperative with their playmates. After watching even a brief episode of TV violence, children may "act out" in more aggressive or hurtful ways. Be aware of what your child watches—and be prepared to say no.

specified period of time. Time out is an effective way of stopping bad behavior because it means the child doesn't receive any reinforcement (such as verbal attention or physical contact) or get any benefits from the inappropriate behavior during the interval. If time out isn't feasible, take away privileges or have the child apologize to the injured party. Physical punishment should be avoided, since it often generates hostility and humiliation in the child. Moreover, it sets an example of aggression at the very time you are trying to teach the child to be nonaggressive.

Conduct Disorders

Many young children are disobedient and at times destructive. In preschool children, conduct problems usually show up as aggressive behavior. In middle childhood, aggressive behavior is still the most common form of antisocial activity but there may also be episodes of stealing, lying, and fire-setting. In adolescence, antisocial activity takes the form of physical aggression, breaking into property and stealing, truancy, drug use, and sexual offences. In the normal child any such behaviors are isolated, short-lived, and mild, and tend to decrease in frequency as the child grows older. In children with conduct disorders, the behavior occurs with greater severity, frequency, and pervasiveness over a variety of settings. The terms "conduct disorder" and "antisocial behavior" are often used synonymously.

How common are conduct disorders?

They are the most prevalent psychopathologic condition of childhood. In a survey of children aged ten and eleven in Britain's Isle of Wight, conduct disorders were diagnosed in 6 percent of the boys and 1.6 percent of the girls. In Ontario, about 5 percent of boys and 2 percent of girls were rated by teachers as showing conduct disorders.

How serious are these disorders?

Children and adolescents with conduct disorders have a higher rate of depression, as well as learning and attentional problems, than other children. They often have specific learning disabilities, particularly reading disorders. (However, most children with learning disabilities do not have conduct disorders.) In spite of having normal intelligence, some of these children have problems with language development and problem solving. Note that poor school performance can lead to low self-esteem and truancy.

How to recognize conduct disorders

A conduct disorder is a negative and persistent pattern of behavior in which the basic rights of others, or the norms or rules appropriate to the child's age, are violated. The disturbance causes significant impairment in the child's social or academic functioning. It's identified by the presence of three or more of the following in the past twelve months, and at least one in the past six months:

Aggression to people and animals

- often bullies, threatens, or intimidates others

- often initiates physical fights

- has used a weapon that can cause serious physical harm to others (such as a bat, brick, knife, or gun)

- has been physically cruel to people

- has been physically cruel to animals

- has stolen while confronting a victim (e.g., mugging, purse snatching)

- has forced someone into sexual activity

Destruction of property

- has deliberately engaged in fire-setting

- has deliberately destroyed someone else's property (other than by fire-setting)

Deceitfulness or theft

- has broken into someone else's house, building, or car

- often lies to obtain goods or favours or to avoid obligations

- has stolen items of non-trivial value without confronting the victim (including forgery and shoplifting)

Serious absences

- often stays out at night against parents' instructions, beginning before age thirteen

- has run away from home overnight at least twice (or once without returning) while living in the parental home, or an equivalent

- has often been truant from school, beginning before age thirteen

Based on Diagnostic and Statistical Manual of Mental Disorders, 4th edition (DSM IV) *of the* American Psychiatric Association

Up to 75 percent of children with conduct disorders also have increased activity levels characteristic of attention deficit–hyperactivity disorder (ADHD). Children with both conduct disorder and ADHD tend to be even more aggressive, and to show a greater variety and severity of antisocial behavior, than children with conduct disorders alone. Children with both disorders are at high risk of continuing their antisocial behavior into adulthood.

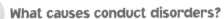

What causes conduct disorders?

The causes are the same as those of aggression in the younger child. There is strong evidence for a genetic influence; a higher than expected rate is found in the children of criminals, and if one identical twin has conduct disorders, the other has a greater than average chance of having them too. Environmental influences have also been shown to be important. Family risk factors such as marital discord and divorce, alcoholism, and psychiatric impairment are known to be associated with antisocial behavior in children. A child whose friends show antisocial behavior is more likely to become involved in this behavior as well.

What can be done about conduct disorders?

A family doctor or pediatrician may be able to counsel the family, but referral to a psychologist or psychiatrist is necessary if the behavior is extreme, unremitting, or violent; if the child's daily functioning is significantly impaired; or if the family can't manage the child. The goal of treatment is to help the child comply with rules appropriate to his or her age, and to decrease the frequency of aggressive behavior.

One of the most effective and best-studied approaches to managing a child with a conduct disorder is training the parents to handle the behavior, as outlined above, in the section "The Aggressive Child." These skills may be learned during therapy sessions and then practiced at home. An alternative treatment is cognitive therapy, in which the child is taught problem-solving skills that can be used in situations that previously might have triggered aggressive behavior. Family therapy has also been used, to establish clear communication and develop mutual negotiating skills, and sometimes family problems accompanying the conduct disorder can be treated at the same time. As well, parents may be advised to improve family relationships, channel the child's energies into positive directions, and improve the child's self-esteem. Marital counseling is sometimes indicated.

Aren't there any medications that help?

Medication plays only a small part in the management of these children. Haloperidol has been used where aggressive outbursts take the form of frequent "blind rages," and Ritalin has been used for ADHD.

Do most children outgrow these problems?

In general, children whose antisocial behavior is limited to minor delinquent acts and who have positive relationships with other children do reasonably well. However, those who have severe antisocial problems and get on poorly with others do not. Long-term studies indicate that 75 percent of children with significant conduct disorders continue their antisocial behavior as adolescents, and 40 to 50 percent have significant problems as adults. These problems include:

- alcoholism and drug abuse;

- increased rate of divorce, separation, and remarriage;

- criminality;

- increased school drop-out rate;

- increased unemployment;

- psychiatric problems, including neuroses and schizophrenia.

Other factors that point to problems in adulthood include conflict in the community as well as at home and in school, and any trouble involving the police.

 Isn't there any way to stop this behavior early?

It's possible that early identification of aggression and other warning signs of conduct disorder may allow these children to be successfully treated. The early signs associated with the development of conduct disorders include:

- aggressive behavior;

- reports that the child is difficult to control;

- hyperactivity;

- oppositional behavior (see below) after age three;

- poor relationships with siblings, including physical aggression, hostility, yelling, and teasing.

The more severe the disorder is at three years of age, the more likely it is to persist to eight years of age. However, if high-risk children are identified, intervention programs may prevent future behavioral problems. These programs should be aimed at helping the child develop social skills, self-control, and self-esteem. Parental programs should be aimed at improving parenting skills and decreasing marital discord.

Oppositional-Defiant Disorder

"Oppositional-defiant disorder" is a term often used with reference to younger children. The disorder includes negativism and hostility but, unlike conduct disorders, not the violation of societal norms. It's characterized by stubbornness, tantrums, disobedience, and defiance of authority. This behavior reaches a peak during the "Terrible Twos" and usually decreases afterwards, but becomes prominent again during the adolescent years.

How to recognize oppositional-defiant disorder

A child is diagnosed as having the disorder only if the problem behavior is considerably more frequent than in most people of the same mental age. The disorder has a pattern of negativistic, hostile, and defiant behavior lasting at least six months, during which four or more of the following are present:

- often loses temper
- often argues with adults
- often actively defies adult requests or rules (e.g., refuses to do chores at home)
- often deliberately does things that annoy other people
- often blames others for mistakes or misbehavior
- is often touchy or easily annoyed
- is often angry and resentful
- is often spiteful or vindictive

Based on Diagnostic and Statistical Manual of Mental Disorders, 4th edition (DSM IV) *of the American Psychiatric Association*

Q What causes oppositional-defiant disorder?

Lax discipline by permissive parents, or unduly harsh, restrictive, or inconsistent discipline, may lead to persistent disobedience in children. Parents who are in stress or conflict, or who show little regard for the law, influence a child's readiness to obey. A very creative or strong-willed child tends to be more stubborn, and a child who is tired, ill, or hungry is less likely to obey.

Q What can I do about oppositional-defiant behavior?

To prevent power struggles between you and your child, allow the child a measure of power over a situation by offering choices; for example, "Do you want to brush your teeth before or after you wash your face?" This allows him or her to learn to solve problems, make decisions, and become more independent. As

173

well, teach the child that when two people can't agree, a compromise allows both to give up a little and still have at least some of what they want. Try to change your position from a demand to a compromise. Use requests and suggestions rather than direct orders. A child who has advance warning, rather than being expected to obey immediately, is more likely to cooperate.

Praise your child when he or she is willing to compromise or cooperate. In addition, use a reward system, such as gold stars on a calendar or coupons to be traded in for future privileges.

Ignore minor defiance, and try to avoid head-to-head combat; instead, teach your child ways to cooperate. It's sometimes necessary to back off from a confrontation or delay a decision, when you're both upset or angry. Remember that even negative attention such as scolding can reinforce a child's misbehavior. Threats are often difficult to carry out, and children soon learn to dismiss them.

Is there any "best way" to make rules?

Tell your child exactly what to do and when it should be done. Instead of saying "Clean up your room," say "Please pick up your toys and make your bed." When you explain the reason for a request, the child may be more willing to comply; for example, add "Then I'll be able to vacuum." Make fewer rules, so they're easier to remember and enforce. State rules in a positive way: that is, tell the child what to do rather than what not to do. Say "Please use your knife and fork" rather than "Don't eat with your fingers." Rules should be enforced consistently, or children will test them at every opportunity. Impose reasonable penalties if rules aren't followed, and avoid excessively harsh punishments, as well as yelling and spanking. A contract that outlines what a teen will do and what a parent will do in return may strengthen the teen's commitment to behave acceptably.

On the whole, a child is more likely to accept your discipline if you have a close relationship with abundant affection. Try to show plenty of love and caring, and spend lots of time with your child. Put up with some signs of rebellion, and let the child win some disagreements that aren't crucial, such as choices of clothes and hairstyles.

Attention Deficit–Hyperactivity Disorder
● ●

Attention deficit–hyperactivity disorder (ADHD) is characterized by inattentiveness, impulsiveness, and hyperactivity, resulting in significantly impaired functioning at home, in school, and/or with peers. In the past, various terms have been used to describe this condition, including "minimal brain damage or dysfunction," "hyperkinesis," "hyperactivity," and "attention-deficit disorder."

About 3 to 5 percent of school-age children have ADHD. It's about six times more frequent in boys than in girls. Symptoms persist into adulthood in 40 to 60 percent of people.

Do children with ADHD always have trouble concentrating?

The symptoms may vary considerably between home and school, structured versus nonstructured settings, large versus small groups, and situations with high versus low performance demands. For example, the child may have difficulty concentrating in monotonous activities but no problem in certain activities of his or her own choice, such as watching TV or playing Nintendo. Most children with ADHD have difficulty concentrating on many activities that other children enjoy, like colouring, pasting, and puzzles. They may also exhibit any of the following: free flight of ideas, difficulty feeling satisfied, social immaturity, inconsistency of performance, and mood swings.

There is now evidence that ADHD *without* hyperactivity, also known as "undifferentiated attention-deficit disorder (UADD)," is a separate disorder. Children with this problem function at a slower cognitive speed and appear more confused, apathetic, and lethargic, and are more likely to be depressed than children with ADHD. They also tend to be identified later, when they begin to fall behind academically in higher primary grades. Children with ADHD are described as being noisier, messier, more disruptive, less responsible, and less mature, and have more problems with peer relationships.

Do children with ADHD have learning disabilities?

Some 25 to 30 percent of these children have a learning disability. Despite having normal, or even superior, intelligence, they are often chronic underachievers. By adolescence up to one-third have failed at least one grade in school.

Many ADHD children have language disorders, most prominent in expressive language. They may have limited vocabularies, difficulties choosing words, and poor grammar. Note that some psychologists feel language development is linked to the development of self-control, as children use inner language to help them monitor their behavior.

Is ADHD associated with psychiatric problems?

As many as 50 to 65 percent of ADHD children have at least one additional psychiatric disorder, often including oppositional-defiant disorder or conduct

How to recognize attention deficit–hyperactivity disorder

This problem appears before the age of seven, creates problems in at least two settings (e.g., at home *and* at school), and causes significant impairment in social or academic functioning. As well, there is impulsiveness and *either* inattention *or* hyperactivity.

Impulsiveness

- often has difficulty awaiting turn in games or group situations

- often blurts out answers to questions before they have been completed

- often interrupts or intrudes on others (e.g., butts into other children's games)

Inattention

Six or more of the following symptoms have persisted for at least six months, to a degree that is maladaptive and inconsistent with the child's level of development:

- often fails to pay close attention to details or makes careless mistakes

- often has difficulty sustaining attention in tasks or play activities

- often doesn't seem to listen when spoken to directly

- often doesn't follow through on instructions, and fails to finish schoolwork or chores (but not due to oppositional behavior or failure to understand)

- often has difficulty organizing tasks and activities

- often avoids, dislikes, or is reluctant to engage in tasks that require sustained mental effort

- often loses things necessary for tasks or activities (e.g., toys, pencils, books, assignments)

- is often easily distracted

- is often forgetful in daily activities

Hyperactivity

Six or more of the following symptoms have persisted for at least six months, to a degree that is maladaptive and inconsistent with the child's level of development:

- often fidgets or squirms in seat

- often leaves seat in classroom or other situations in which remaining seated is expected

- often runs about or climbs excessively in inappropriate situations (in adolescents this may be limited to feelings of restlessness)

- often has difficulty playing or engaging in leisure activities quietly

- often talks excessively

- is often "on the go" or acts as if "driven by a motor"

Based on Diagnostic and Statistical Manual of Mental Disorders, 4th edition (DSM IV) *of the American Psychiatric Association* disorder. Those who come from dysfunctional families with alcoholism, drug abuse, and violence are most at risk of developing serious antisocial behavior during adolescence.

Problems with poor self-esteem are common, and 25 to 33 percent of ADHD children experience at least one episode of major depression during their childhood years. Anxiety disorders resulting in fears and worries also occur in up to 25 percent of ADHD children.

What causes ADHD?

The cause is unknown, but there is evidence that the frontal lobes of the brain may be involved; they have long been known to play a critical role in regulating attention, activity, and emotional reactions. Studies have shown decreased blood flow in the frontal areas of children with ADHD. As well, PET (positive emission tomography) scans have shown that adults with ADHD have reduced brain glucose metabolism in the frontal lobes of the brain when they try to concentrate on a task. This pattern of underactivity may be due to abnormalities in the neurotransmitters (chemical messengers) in the frontal areas. It has been suggested that stimulant medication may compensate for such abnormalities, since ADHD subjects show increased activity in these frontal areas when treated with such medications.

Heredity plays a role in ADHD, since ADHD children are four times more likely to have close family members with the same problem. Also, identical twins are more likely to share ADHD than are fraternal twins or other siblings.

Birth injuries associated with fetal distress and difficult labor play a negligible role, but damage *prior* to birth may be a factor. Mothers who abuse drugs or alcohol during pregnancy have more children who suffer from ADHD and learning disabilities.

Environmental toxins, including lead, and artificial flavors, dyes, preservatives, and other food additives, have been claimed by some to be the primary cause of ADHD. Some doctors claim that sugar, food allergy, and food additives cause ADHD, and use anecdotal evidence and testimonials to back up their claims. "Double-blind" controlled studies (in which neither the subjects nor the researchers know what substance is being administered) have shown that these are *not* important causes. It's true that recent research has shown that in a select group of children, food allergies and sensitivities to food dyes may contribute to behavioral problems and physical symptoms, although no differences were noticed in psychological test scores. Some of these studies involved preschool children with ADHD and known allergies

177

or sensitivities, and avoidance of the triggers resulted in improved behavior as well as fewer problems with headaches, runny noses, and sleep. But these children were not representative of ADHD children in general.

How is ADHD diagnosed?

There's no single test that gives a definitive diagnosis. A history of long-standing problems of attention, impulsiveness, and hyperactivity is the best source of clues. Of course, the parents will supply one account. Because symptoms may vary with the situation, the physician should also obtain reports from teachers concerning the child's ability to finish work, stay on task, and respect the fact that others are important. Given the association of ADHD and learning difficulties, the teachers' reports may help in assessing the level of academic achievement and general intelligence. In many cases, behavioral therapies and medication (see below) result in significant improvement in behavior and school performance. If not, referral to other specialists may be necessary. A referral to an educational psychologist may be necessary to exclude learning disabilities. Speech and language assessment may be necessary if a communication problem is suspected. Examination of the child's emotional status may be necessary to rule out depression and anxiety disorders, and to distinguish ADHD from other disruptive behavior problems such as conduct disorders and oppositional-defiant disorder. A medical examination is necessary to rule out visual and hearing problems, because attention and memory may be further impaired by any sensory deficits.

Various rating scales have been used to assess behavior at home and in school. The Conners Teacher Rating Scale rates children on several aspects of behavior, as does the ADDH Comprehensive Teacher Rating Scale (ACTeRS), which allows for separate evaluation of four areas of behavior. These scales are helpful in making an initial diagnosis and in monitoring the child's response to treatment. There are also performance tests to assess the child's ability to sustain and focus attention, as well as his or her ability to refrain from responding impulsively. These include the Matching Familiar Figures Test and the Continuous Performance Test. While these tests provide useful information, the results are not infallible, and should be interpreted in the context of all available information.

What can be done about ADHD?

The goals of therapy are to improve the child's functioning at home, in school, and with other children, through modifying his or her inattention, impulsiveness, and hyperactivity. In addition there is an attempt to improve cognitive functioning, social and behavior skills, and self-esteem as far as possible with minimal side effects. The long-term outcome of ADHD has been shown to improve most with a combination of parental education, medication, psychological treatments, and appropriate classroom intervention.

How do I educate myself about ADHD?

The first step is to obtain comprehensive, accurate information about ADHD, associated problems, and treatments from your doctor. Support groups such as CHADD (Children and Adults with Attention Deficit Disorders) and ADDA (Attention Deficit Disorders Association) also provide important educational and support services, and give parents a forum in which to discuss problems, provide emotional support, and share effective ways to deal with schools, doctors, and service institutions.

What kinds of medication are used for ADHD?

Stimulants and tricyclic antidepressants are commonly used, and clonidine, a blood-pressure medication, may also be helpful.

Stimulants such as Ritalin (most commonly used), Dexedrine, and Pemoline are the first choice. Numerous studies have shown that they are effective in more than 70 percent of ADHD children. Some 70 percent of those children who do not respond to one of these will respond to a second. Stimulants don't sedate ADHD children, but help them focus their attention, control their impulsive behavior, and regulate their activity level. Stimulants are felt to act as neurotransmitters in certain areas of the brain, correcting a biochemical condition that interferes with attention and impulse control. Often there is a noticeable change in handwriting, talking, attention, inappropriate activity, compliance, and academic performance within just one hour of starting treatment.

Many studies have shown stimulant medications to be quite safe, and side effects are minimal and mild. Those most commonly seen are insomnia, loss of appetite, and weight loss. Less common side effects include sadness, depression, fearfulness, social withdrawal, sleepiness, headaches, nail biting, and stomach aches. All side effects are short-term, and the majority disappear if the drug dosage is lowered. Long-term studies have found that children treated with stimulants do not become addicted, and the medication does not lead to illegal drug use in later years. Studies have also shown that while stimulants may cause some suppression of growth during the first year or two of treatment, this is a transient problem and the effect on adult height is minimal. Stimulant drugs are also effective in adolescents, and the dosage is the same as for older children.

Tricyclic antidepressants, such as imipramine and desipramine, also produce improvement in more than 70 percent of ADHD children. The improvements in behavior are usually more prominent than the improvements in attention. It is felt that tricyclics also act as neurotransmitters, but work by improving the child's mood, impulsiveness, and tolerance of frustration.

Common side effects include dry mouth, constipation, and drowsiness. Rarely, irregularities of heart rhythm have been reported in children taking tricyclics, so it may be necessary to have an electrocardiogram (EKG) done by a physician. Tricyclics are generally used as a second line of drug therapy, for children who don't benefit from Ritalin or who develop side effects on stimulant medication. Ritalin is the first drug of choice for those who have depression or anxiety associated with ADHD. It may also be used in children with ADHD who have tics or Tourette's syndrome (a disorder causing abnormal speech and movement). Tricyclics should never be discontinued abruptly; the dosage should be tapered off.

Clonidine, a blood-pressure medication, has been found to decrease overactivity, aggression, and impulsiveness in about 50 percent of ADHD children. It doesn't improve distractibility, but may be used in combination with Ritalin. Clonidine takes about two weeks to cause any improvement, and its most common side effect is drowsiness, usually short-lived. Like tricyclics, clonidine should never be discontinued abruptly.

 What kind of psychological treatments are used for ADHD?
A number of psychological and behavioral therapies, alone or in combination, have been used with varying degrees of success. The aim is to modify the associated problems, such as oppositional-defiant behavior and conduct problems.

Parental training provides a variety of management strategies for the behavioral problems seen in ADHD children. Problems such as noncompliance, defiance, and aggression are treated by the methods outlined above for the oppositional-defiant and aggressive child. This training can be offered to individuals or to groups, and involves direct instruction, modeling, role-playing, and discussion. It has been shown to be moderately effective in helping parents manage and change behavior in ADHD children.

Family therapy deals with a variety of approaches to family-skills training, including problem solving, open and effective communication skills, anger management, and conflict resolution.

Classroom management uses procedures similar to the strategies parents learn in parental training (e.g., praise and reinforcement and aggression management). Many well-conducted studies have proved that this improves classroom behavior and academic performance. The ideal class for the ADHD child is highly structured and well organized, with clear expectations and a predictable schedule. The child should be seated near the teacher, and away from windows and other distractions. Because the child works slowly, he or she should be allowed extra time to complete tests and assignments. The amount of written work may be reduced until the child is better able to cope. A daily homework planner helps the child develop organizational and time-management skills. Communication between parents and teachers is important so that academic progress can be monitored.

Problem-solving training attempts to help ADHD children deal with impulsive behavior. The children are taught to solve problems by saying to themselves, "Stop, decide possible plans of action, do the plan, evaluate the success of the plan." Both parents and teachers must help by modeling, promoting, and encouraging the use of problem solving. Used alone, this type of training is not as effective as stimulant therapy or behavior-modification programs.

Anger-management training aims to teach the child to recognize anger signals, and to use techniques like relaxation methods and coping statements to deal with the anger.

Group social-skills training is helpful for children who have poor social skills and have trouble relating to others their own age. They are taught practical techniques such as maintaining eye contact, initiating and maintaining conversation, and cooperating.

Academic intervention, in the form of individual remedial education, may be needed for children who have learning disabilities. Parents and educators work together to decide on the best classroom placement for these children. This process is generally carried out through an Individual Placement and Review Committee at the child's school.

Non-standard therapies of many kinds have been tried for ADHD and learning disorders. Although few of these treatments are harmful, most have not been proven to have any benefit. "Orthomolecular" therapies include the use of megavitamins and essential fatty acids and various restrictive diets (allergy-free, yeast-free, sucrose-restricted, salicylate-free). "Neurophysiologic" therapies include alpha-wave conditioning, patterning, sensory-integration training, optometric training, eye-muscle exercises, and tinted lenses. Other approaches include therapy against motion sickness, and chiropractic manipulation.

None of these has been shown to be effective in double-blind controlled clinical trials.

What happens when ADHD children grow up?

Long-term studies have shown that 40 to 60 percent of children who have ADHD still have symptoms in adulthood. Untreated adults are more likely to have aggressive behavior, antisocial personality disorder, conduct disorder, depression, divorce, school drop-out, and alcohol and drug abuse. Adult ADHD is now being recognized more frequently, and treated with medications similar to those used for children.

Learning Disabilities

"Learning disabilities" (LD) is a term that refers to a varied group of disorders that show up as significant difficulties in listening, speaking, reading, spelling, writing, reasoning, and/or mathematics. These disorders are not due to environmental factors and are presumed to be caused by dysfunction of the central nervous system. The term does *not* apply to children whose learning problems are primarily the result of visual, hearing, or motor handicaps; mental retardation; emotional disturbance; or environmental, cultural, or economic disadvantage. Most children with LD have average or above average intelligence.

What are the signs of a learning disability?

Currently, the most accepted indication of a learning disability is a significant discrepancy between a child's potential for learning and his or her achievement. Children with LD have difficulties learning in the traditional way at the accepted rate for their age group. For some reason their channels for learning don't process stimuli in the usual way. As a result, both understanding and expression can be affected. The Learning Disabilities Association of Canada says 10 percent of Canadians have a learning disability serious enough to require some form of therapy. Learning disabilities affect boys and girls equally, although more boys are referred for help, perhaps because they are more disruptive to parents and teachers.

Learning problems can be divided into two main groups:

- involvement of auditory visual processes, resulting in reading disorders (dyslexia) and other language-based learning problems;

- involvement of visual and motor processes (nonverbal learning disabilities, or NLD), resulting in poor handwriting (dysgraphia), problems with mathematics (dyscalculia), and below-average social skills.

What causes dyslexia?

Dyslexia is the most common learning disability, and the one that creates the most long-term problems. It's caused not by a vision problem but by impaired language-processing skills. Dyslexics have a problem decoding "phonemes," the individual speech sounds in the alphabet, and have difficulty with "phonics," the ability to sound out words. As a result, they have trouble reading the letters of the alphabet, and so can't concentrate on the meaning of the words.

Dyslexics also have a problem with verbal short-term memory, and therefore have problems recalling letters, words, phrases, names, dates, phone numbers, addresses, and rote facts. Besides having problems with understanding written material, many of those with auditory processing problems have difficulty understanding what they hear; they may confuse words like "dog" and "log," especially in a noisy environment. They may have trouble following verbal instructions.

Another problem for dyslexics is mathematics, because they have difficulty memorizing basic math facts and remembering sequences of steps. They often reverse or mislabel numbers (e.g., 13 for 30), and often have difficulty understanding written math problems. Dyslexics often have a history of delayed speech, and of mispronouncing words; certain sounds are omitted, substituted, or distorted.

What happens in nonverbal learning disabilities (NLDs)?

NLDs constitute about 1 to 10 percent of all learning disabilities. Problems with arithmetic and handwriting, as well as social awareness and social judgment, are associated with NLD. The right side of the brain processes nonverbal information and deals with spatial awareness, recognition of visual patterns, and coordination of visual information with motor processes (visual-motor integration). Children with NLD can have psychomotor and tactile-perceptual deficits and may be poorly coordinated in gross and fine motor skills. As a result, they are late learning to tie shoes, hold a pencil, catch a ball, ride a bike, and assemble puzzles. They have visual-perceptual-organizational deficits and have problems with exercises in eye-hand coordination such as handwriting, drawing, and copying from the blackboard.

In mathematics they have trouble understanding fundamental concepts, or what approach they should use to solve a problem. They may, however, have strong psycholinguistic skills such as rote verbal learning, word recognition, and spelling.

These children are often described as being isolated, with few close friends and limited social activity. They have problems understanding jokes, game strategies, the motives of others, and social conventions. They often lack insight into their own future, and their strengths and weaknesses. Possible reasons for these problems include poor social comprehension, inability to imagine the perspective of others, misinterpretation of body language, impulsiveness, and being easily led.

Are these various disorders ever combined?

ADHD occurs in 26 to 41 percent of children with learning disabilities. This combination may be due to the fact that ADHD children are inattentive and learn poorly, or "tune out"—or perhaps some children with LD are unable to keep paying attention because the academic demands made on them are too hard, and they feel frustrated. Studies suggest that ADHD and LD are *not* genetically linked.

Depression and anxiety disorders occur in one-third of LD children, especially those with nonverbal learning disabilities. It's not surprising, since these children often have very low levels of self-esteem after years of failing at school and being labeled "stupid" by their peers.

What causes learning disabilities?

Heredity is a primary factor in language-based learning disabilities. As with ADHD, there is a link between learning disabilities and maternal abuse of alcohol and cocaine during pregnancy. Dyslexia is associated with dysfunction on the left side of the brain, the side specialized for language. Researchers have found that an area in the left hemisphere known as the *planum temporale*, which is normally larger on the left side than on the right, is either the same size or smaller in dyslexics.

Nonverbal learning disabilities have been found in children with severe head injuries, hydrocephalus (too much fluid within the skull), and radiation treatment of the head. Since these conditions involve destruction of white matter in the right hemisphere, it's felt that NLDs are caused by early damage to this white matter.

How are learning disabilities diagnosed?

It's important that a diagnosis be made before skill levels and self-esteem slip to dangerous lows. The child's physician should look for any neurological dysfunction and assess hearing and vision to rule out sensory or neurological problems affecting learning. The doctor should also take a history of developmental milestones to rule out mental retardation and autism and ask about behavior and attention span. Medications such as antihistamines, anticonvulsants, tranquillizers, and asthma drugs can affect attention and learning. Formal assessment of intelligence and educational achievement by a psychologist is occasionally necessary. Reports from teachers and/or IQ tests can give information about the child's cognitive strengths and weaknesses, and may help define how well the child processes information. Some of the more frequently used intelligence tests for school-age children are the Wechsler Intelligence Scale for Children (WISC-III) and the Stanford-Binet Intelligence Scale. Academic achievement can be assessed by tests such as the Peabody Individual Achievement Test–Revised (PIAT–R), the Woodcock-Johnson Tests of Achievement–Revised (W-J–R), and the Wide Range Achievement Test–Revised (WRAT–R).

What can be done about learning disabilities?

The cornerstone of treatment is educational therapy, tailored to the child's individual needs and depending on his or her learning strengths and weaknesses. There are many programs to teach reading skills, including intensive phonetic teaching programs.

Besides remedial reading techniques, some teachers have tried instructing LD children in learning strategies. There has been some success in teaching them to improve the way they approach new tasks, memorize new information (such as using mnemonics), and organize information (such as using rhymes or visual images to link bits of information together). One successful strategy is the "write–say" method, in which the student rewrites incorrectly spelled words several times while spelling the words out loud. A variant of this method has proved successful in teaching multiplication tables.

Other methods of helping LD children include having other children in the class or school act as tutors, and using computer-assisted instruction. Children with writing disorders may be helped by homework buddies, oral testing, using a classmate's notes, and being taught keyboarding.

Social-skills training, psychological counseling, and behavior-management techniques are often used, but have not been shown to be consistently helpful. In the child with LD and ADHD, stimulant medications have been shown to improve classroom performance, not only through improved attentiveness, but also in the way the central nervous system processes information. In reading tasks, this effect is seen in improved word-finding abilities.

Most boards of education are required by law to provide specialized education for LD children. This may mean special classes, special teachers, or even a special school. There is evidence, though, that teaching LD students in regular classes, using highly motivated, well-trained teachers and teachers' aides, can lead to improvements in academic performance, behavior, and self-esteem.

Where can I get more detailed information about LD children?

One of the most valuable supports for parents is the Association for Children with Learning Disabilities (ACLD). It provides parents with information about local services and new discoveries, and offers support groups in which parents can compare notes and encourage each other. For more information on this and other groups mentioned, see "Further Resources," at the end of the book.

What happens when LD children grow up?

Most children with reading disability can compensate and attain literacy, but as adults they may do less well in work as well as in social and psychological adjustment. The outcome is better for those who are of higher intelligence, have a less severe disability, are in a higher socio-economic class, attend private school, are not hyperactive, and have no known neurological problems. With the right support systems, many people with LD achieve high academic and professional success; two good examples are Winston Churchill and Thomas Edison.

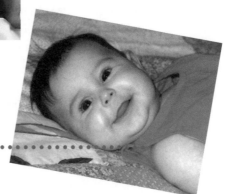

CHAPTER 16

The Child with Chronic Pain

●●

There are few problems more distressing to parents than seeing their own child in pain. None of us wants to see our children suffer, and our instinctive reaction is to do our utmost to bring relief from the pain. Usually we think of pain as a sudden, acute sign of potentially serious problem that needs immediate attention: an accidental knife cut, a sprained ankle, acute appendicitis.

Not all pain is like that. "Chronic" pains tend to occur over and over again, sometimes in predictable patterns. The problems considered here are familiar to many experienced parents, and include recurrent stomachaches, headaches, teething pains, growing pains, and others.

Q How can I tell if my child's pain is serious?

Unlike that for acute pain, the time frame for many chronic-pain problems may be weeks, months, or even years. The child may not be obviously unwell, but may have been complaining about the same symptoms for a very long time. Parents might be ready to accept similar symptoms in themselves or another adult, but in the case of their children they worry that some major problem is being overlooked. Their fears may grow worse if they hear stories from other parents or relatives about someone's illness being missed or misdiagnosed. On occasion, parents are convinced that there must be something wrong simply because the complaints have lasted so long. In fact, the reverse is often true: the shorter the duration, the more likely it is that the pain is due to an illness or abnormality—although time alone is not a reliable way to judge the cause or seriousness of pain.

Most of the situations outlined below are common in childhood, and most can be dealt with by parents without much medical intervention.

However, there are always exceptions, and each child needs to be considered individually. No written advice (not even this chapter!) can substitute for careful assessment of the child's problems. This chapter is written in the hope of helping you understand some chronic-pain scenarios—*not* as a specific aid to diagnosis.

Recurrent Abdominal Pain

"Recurrent abdominal pain" (RAP) is the name commonly used to describe the symptoms of children who complain of repeated episodes of stomachache or pain. From 5 to 10 percent of children experience RAP at one time or another. It's so frequently seen by pediatricians that it has been a subject of study in pediatric journals for decades. Each year there are new theories about the cause, and each idea rides a wave of popularity for a while. Causes suggested in both the medical and lay press in recent years include:

- *lactose intolerance*—an inability to digest the sugar commonly contained in milk and milk products, resulting in gas, cramps, and sometimes diarrhea (see Chapter 12, "Feeding Your Child");

- *gastroesophageal reflux*—regurgitation of acid from the stomach upwards into the esophagus (swallowing tube), sometimes causing a sensation of pain or "heartburn" (see Chapter 7, "Spitting Up, Vomiting, and Diarrhea");

- *H. pylori infection*—ulceration and inflammation caused by *H. pylori*, a bacteria that lives in the stomach. While this can occur in children, and can cause pain, there are also studies showing that it can occur just as frequently in children without pain. It may be *a* cause, but it's certainly not *the* cause;

- *food allergy*—a convenient diagnosis for a wide variety of problems that don't have an easy solution. It's wise to be sceptical. If there is not a clear and obvious reaction to a specific food each time it's consumed, it's unlikely to be the culprit, no matter what the allergy tests may show (see Chapter 12).

How can I tell what's causing my child's abdominal pain?

The vast majority of children with this problem will never be diagnosed with a "disease" related to it. Nevertheless, there are several factors that may contribute to the situation, and you should consider all of them.

Start with the question of language. Most children don't willingly describe the pain; they usually say, "My tummy hurts," and *we* interpret that as a statement of pain. In fact, very young children use the expression "hurts" to describe any sensation outside their usual range of experience. Try suggesting that the child go to the bathroom as a first step in relieving a "tummyache"; the sensation that adults recognize as a need to pass a bowel movement may well be a "hurt" to a young child. Similarly, they may say "hurts" to describe a variety of other sensations, including nausea, nervousness or "butterflies," hunger, a full feeling after a meal, mild cramps, or the need to urinate. Depending on the nature of your response, this descriptive pattern may become ingrained, and may remain part of the child's vocabulary in later years.

Parents can be good detectives if they look for other clues to the significance of the pain. By using examples the child recognizes, you may be able to narrow down the problem. For example, "Does it feel like you have to throw up? Does it feel like you have to poop or pee? Does it feel like you ate too much?" A good detective is also a good observer. Note the time pattern of recurrent pain (just before leaving for school, just before bedtime, or after meals, for example), and see how the child looks when he or she complains. Sometimes a child talks about pain in a very matter-of-fact manner, and a few minutes later goes out to play. It's particularly important to see how much the pain interferes with activities the child enjoys (playing with friends, etc.), as opposed to those he or she may not enjoy (such as school).

RAP is often associated with constipation. Sometimes the problem is evident; the child simply doesn't have a bowel movement very often. But there are also children whose constipation is less apparent; they seem to move their bowels daily, but they still have a lot of stool backed up in the bowel, causing frequent cramps. Studies have shown that many of these children get pain relief when fiber is added to their diets, even though they've never complained of constipation. Occasionally, children develop patterns of stool-withholding that may be difficult for them to change on their own. These children tend to have a large accumulation of stool in the large bowel, and may pass a bowel movement in the toilet only once every few days. The movements tend to be very large. In between, they may have "accidents," soiling their underwear with stool that seeps down past the accumulation in the rectum. This problem, called "encopresis," may also cause cramps and complaints of abdominal pain. (See Chapter 6, "Toilet Training.")

Events in the child's environment (home, family, and school) may also be factors in recurrent abdominal pain. Children tend to be creatures of habit, and major changes in their world can be quite disruptive. Some express their upset or anxiety in words, but others show the stress through a variety of physical symptoms, including abdominal pain. Moving, resulting in a change in city, home, and/or school, is disturbing to many children. The death of a relative, or even a pet, is difficult for them to understand and may trigger problems. The birth of a baby brother or sister is almost guaranteed to produce some degree of jealousy (in other words, it's normal), but may have a greater impact on some children. Finally, tensions within the home, especially marital difficulty, virtually always affect children to some degree.

Although it may seem hard to believe, abdominal pain can actually be rewarding to some children. Being ill usually attracts parental concern and attention, which sometimes reinforces a pattern of behavior that may have started quite innocently. When the parents are separated, a child's illness is often the only thing that will bring the pair together around the child.

Is abdominal pain ever hereditary?

In thinking about your child's pain, also take a close look at yourself. Parents with chronic abdominal problems are more likely to have children with RAP. Some adults have intestinal symptoms on a regular basis without necessarily having a disease. Do you have irritable-bowel syndrome? Do you get diarrhea whenever you're nervous or upset? Do you have a sensitive stomach? Do you vomit more easily than most people? Do you have problems with chronic constipation? A "yes" to any of these questions may indicate that the pattern runs in the family. In other words, the apple doesn't usually fall far from the tree! The situation may be intensified by the fact that adults who have these problems tend to focus on them, and may talk about them in front of their children, so that the children have considerable exposure to the issues during their formative years.

You should also take a close look at your own concerns and anxiety. If a relative has recently died of stomach cancer, for example, you may be particularly worried about stomach pain in your child. While there's no reason to suppose there's any link between the two, the worry is understandable. By recognizing the source of your concern, you may be able to keep it in perspective, and avoid increasing your child's anxiety. Admit your concern to the physician; it's likely that the disease you fear can be easily ruled out.

How often is abdominal pain a sign of serious disease?

Obviously, not all recurrent abdominal pain can be attributed to the causes and circumstances above. Pediatric textbooks contain literally hundreds of causes of such pain. However, those hundreds of causes account for about 5 percent of all the children who have this symptom. For the remaining 95 percent, no obvious disease is found.

Understandably, no parent wants his or her child to be part of the 5 percent with a disease, and many parents push for tests to rule out serious illness. Unfortunately, children are frequently overtested for this reason. Testing for the sake of "ruling out," in the absence of any evidence to suggest a particular diagnosis, is rarely helpful. Often it does more harm than good, by inflicting procedures that make the child feel even more ill and vulnerable. It's far more valuable to spend time reviewing the issues listed above than to go on a "fishing expedition" of laboratory tests and X rays.

 What if no serious illness is found?

If your child belongs to the 95 percent whose pain can't be related to a specific disease, you should be relieved; that's usually better than the alternative. If you find this conclusion difficult to accept, and fear that something may have been overlooked, it's important that you feel comfortable enough with your doctor to ask questions until all your concerns have been answered.

Even more important, don't assume that your child is "making up" the symptoms. Pain is a very subjective sensation, and we all learn different thresholds (tolerances) for pain as we grow up. The abdominal discomfort may be very real to the child even though no disease is involved. After all, an adult who develops diarrhea when nervous, or who becomes nauseated at the sight of blood, isn't "making up" these symptoms, yet they aren't related to disease. They are just examples of how closely the stomach and intestines are linked to the brain and emotions—in both adults and children.

When abdominal pain is important

There are a few circumstances that do call for prompt medical assessment. If your child's recurrent abdominal pain is associated with weight loss, recurrent fevers, chronic diarrhea, blood in the stools, pain or difficulty with urination, or frequent vomiting, you should certainly see a physician. The location of the pain may also be noteworthy. Usually, children point to their navels as the site of pain; if the pain is persistently on one side, or if it's felt in the back, further assessment is usually appropriate.

In the absence of specific illness, what can you do to help your child? Details depend on the situation, but here are some general tips that may be helpful.

- Don't ask about pain if the child hasn't brought the subject up, and never ask if he or she had any pain today. If you do, most children will say yes; if you don't, the child may not mention it. You can be sure that if the pain is significant, the child will refer to it. If the subject isn't discussed, the pattern is less likely to be reinforced and may ultimately disappear.

- Teach the child ways to deal with the discomfort without disrupting the rest of the household. He or she may want to go to the bathroom, and then perhaps lie down in the bedroom for a little while until the feeling passes. (Similarly, it's preferable that the child lie down for a few minutes in the school nurse's office rather than come home.)

- If psychological or social stresses may be playing a role (the death of a relative, a recent move, marital problems), they need to be dealt with openly. Professional counseling may be appropriate. Note that the focus of the counseling needn't be the abdominal pain, but rather the stresses that underlie it.

- Display an attitude of understanding and empathy, while encouraging your child to participate in normal routines as far as possible. School attendance is particularly important.

- Avoid extremes in dietary habits, and try to maintain regular mealtimes. While most recurrent abdominal pain is not due to food allergy or intolerance, some children are sensitive to excesses in their diet. For example, those who drink huge amounts of fruit juice each day, especially apple juice, may have abdominal discomfort. By the same token, adding a little fiber to the diet—in the form of whole wheat bread, popcorn, fiber cereals, or high-fiber cookies—may reduce the symptoms.

Growing Pains

It's not at all clear how "growing pains" got their name. There's no real evidence that they have anything to do with growing, except that they seem to occur exclusively at an age when children are growing rapidly. The term refers to pains in the legs; although there's no clear explanation for them, they are indeed real. Furthermore, they have some characteristics that are common enough to be very helpful in establishing a diagnosis.

Typically, these pains occur in children between the ages of three and ten years, particularly towards the younger end of that range. They usually come at night, often while the child is in bed, and seem to affect mainly the lower legs, especially the knees and shins. In most cases it's not difficult to distinguish growing pains from other, potentially serious problems in the legs. Here are some hints.

- Growing pains generally affect both legs. An injury or other abnormality is more likely to involve one leg, not both.

- The pain often comes when the child is motionless and not putting weight on the legs. In almost any other problem of bone, joint, or muscle, the pain is worse when the affected part is in use, or at least bearing weight.

- The child gets relief from someone rubbing or massaging the affected area. A child with a sore joint or a bruise doesn't like to have the area touched.

- Once asleep, the child rarely awakens until morning, and at that time is usually fine. More serious problems are unlikely to resolve that quickly.

- If the child limps, growing pains are very unlikely to be the cause. Consult your child's physician.

What can be done about growing pains?

As with most problems in childhood, there's a wide spectrum of severity. Most children have a pattern that's easily recognizable and doesn't need any investigation. A few have pain that is not typical and may be unusually bad. These children may benefit from a referral to a physician experienced with such problems, and may require some tests before a diagnosis can be made. There is no test for typical growing pains, however. The diagnosis is made by recognizing the classic pattern, and by checking that there's no evidence to suggest any other cause.

Treatment tends to be simple. A pain reliever such as acetaminophen may provide relief at bedtime. (ASA should be used with caution in children; see the remarks on Reye's syndrome in Chapter 5, "Fever.") Massage of the area, or application of heat, may also be helpful.

Teething Pain

Does teething cause pain? It may seem like heresy even to ask such a question, since generations of parents have been absolutely convinced that it does. Teething has also been alleged to cause fever, rash, diarrhea, and vomiting in young infants. Yet, despite the fact that teething is a universal phenomenon, there's not a shred of reliable evidence that it plays a role in any of these common childhood problems!

The many beliefs about teething are not unique to North America. In many cultures, teething is seen as a disease requiring specific intervention and treatment. Is it conceivable that millions of parents, grandparents, and great-grandparents could be wrong? Let's consider some facts.

From the time they're born, newborns are continually exposed to a variety of common viruses, carried by adult caregivers and siblings who may not, themselves, be ill. The most common signs of illness when infants are infected with such viruses are fever, rash, and diarrhea—the same signs attributed to teething. Why, then, does teething get the blame? The usual sequence of events is as follows: A parent notes that the infant is warm, has a rash, or has diarrhea; the parent then looks in the baby's mouth, and specifically at the gums; from about 3 to 4 months of age until 2½ years of age, there is virtually *always* a tooth in the process of erupting. As soon as the parent sees the swollen gum, he or she assumes that the diagnosis has been made. But if the parent looked at the gums on a day when the baby had no symptoms, he or she would probably see a very similar picture!

Surely teething must cause some pain?

It may be reasonable to assume that the little bit of swelling and redness observed over the gum just before the tooth breaks through involves slight discomfort, but there's no logical way to connect this to the other symptoms described above. Even when babies drool and put things in their mouths, it's not clear whether this is because of gum pain or is simply part of normal development. After all, some normal children don't show a tooth until twelve months of age, but they still start putting things in their mouths at four to five months.

The danger of blaming illnesses on teething is that it may prevent us from looking for the real cause. While most fevers are due to viruses that will get better on their own, without treatment, occasionally an infant develops a more dangerous infection. With very young babies it can be difficult to tell the difference between minor and major illnesses, and assessment by an experienced physician may be very important.

Since teething isn't a disease, does it require treatment?

There's no shortage of teething preparations in any drugstore, but in general it's wise to avoid them. There have been rare instances of children suffering serious side effects when such medicines were improperly used, or when they got into the wrong hands (such as a two-year-old eating an entire tube of teething gel). While such incidents may not be likely, it hardly seems worth taking chances just to treat a "non-disease." After all, what could be more normal than a healthy baby growing teeth? It's just part of human growth, and we should treat it as such.

Headache

Like abdominal pain, headache tends to be a recurrent phenomenon in some children. Although many parents have the idea that children shouldn't get headaches, they are in fact quite common, especially in school-age and adolescent children. A headache is frequently part of a viral illness in a child, as it is with an adult; this situation can often be recognized by fever and other accompanying symptoms, such as a sore throat and swollen glands.

Why do some children get headaches if they're not sick?

Simply put, some children are headache-prone. Often at least one of the parents has the same problem. The pattern of recurrent headaches may develop at a fairly young age, but is more likely to start after children are in school. The children are otherwise healthy and function normally in every way. The most common cause of the headache is migraine, which also tends to run in families.

What happens in migraine?

Migraine is best understood as a change in the size of the blood vessels that carry blood to the brain. Arteries, being lined by muscle, have the ability to

---

Headaches and brain tumours

The underlying fear of every parent whose child has headaches is that there may be an ominous problem causing them, and a brain tumour is the worst fear; although parents rarely mention the possibility, they usually acknowledge having thought about it. But brain tumours are among the *rarest* causes of headaches in children. When they are the cause, they characteristically produce a pattern of early-morning headache and vomiting, and the headache itself may gradually become unrelenting. Any child whose headache is associated with early-morning vomiting, seizures, difficulty with speech or movement, or a change in consciousness should obviously be seen by a physician as soon as possible.

become narrow or wider. In migraine headache, the arteries first constrict (become tighter), sometimes causing symptoms such as visual disturbances or "funny feelings," and then dilate (become wider). When they dilate, the headache usually begins.

Children with migraine often feel nauseated, and may even vomit. They frequently like to avoid bright light and loud noises, and may be most comfortable if they lie down in a dark room and try to sleep. Migraine may be triggered by fatigue, exercise, or long periods in the sun. Also, food triggers can sometimes be identified, and it may be valuable to keep a record of what was eaten just prior to a headache, to see if a pattern emerges. Common culprits include nuts, caffeine (as in cola drinks), and spiced meats, among others. With time, both parents and children become expert in identifying the pattern of migraine. They can usually tell when an episode is beginning, and they know what to do.

Q What can I do for a child with migraine?

Most children with migraine can be treated with the simple measures listed above, and with acetaminophen. Note that it's important to give medication as early as possible. In an effort to avoid using medicine unnecessarily, parents sometimes wait to see if the headache will disappear on its own. The longer a migraine headache has been present, the more difficult it is to get rid of. Therefore, once you are familiar with your child's migraine pattern, treat it early rather than late. Be sure that school staff also know how to proceed.

Some migraine is particularly troublesome and doesn't respond to these simple measures. If so, consultation with a physician is strongly advised.

Q What else can cause headaches in children?

Tension headaches are the other major cause. While they are more common in adolescents, they can occur in preteens as well. These headaches produce a sense of tightness around the head, especially over the temples. The neck muscles may also be tight.

Typically, tension headaches are a response to stress. Most of us have experienced them at one time or another—after a particularly difficult day at work or an emotionally draining event at home. Children and teens are no different in their responses to stress; the challenge may be to find out what the stress is. Indeed, the children themselves may not recognize the stresses affecting them.

If children aren't willing to talk openly about these issues with their parents (sometimes because the home environment is part of the problem), professional help may be necessary. As a first step, the problem should be discussed with the family doctor or pediatrician. A referral to a psychologist or psychiatrist may be recommended. With such expert help it should be possible to understand the underlying issues; also, many psychologists can teach the child methods of self-relaxation to help relieve the headaches. A child who gains more control of what happens to his or her body will be less vulnerable to headaches.

Chest Pain

Chest pain is not very common in children, and it always frightens parents, probably because they have been warned to think of it as an early sign of a heart attack. In children, heart problems very seldom cause chest pain. In fact, even in children who are born with heart abnormalities, chest pain is quite rare.

 How do you find the cause of a child's chest pain?

In most cases, tests are not very helpful. The story of the pain is far more useful; by asking the right questions, an experienced doctor can often decide whether or not X rays or other tests need to be done. Even anxiety and depression can cause chest pain, and in these cases it's more important to find the cause of the problem than to provide pain medication.

The commonest cause of chest pain in children is "musculoskeletal," meaning that it comes from muscle or bone. The entire chest wall is lined with muscles (they help you breathe), and a cramp or spasm in one of the muscles can cause a sharp pain, especially when the child takes a deep breath. (Some people call this a "stitch.") Some children and adolescents are particularly prone to this. Also, just as muscles in the leg can get sore or pulled from overuse, so can muscles in the chest. A child with a violent cough may eventually develop chest pain from all the strain, although this usually improves as the cough gets better.

"Heartburn," another cause of chest pain, has nothing to do with the heart. It is essentially the same problem as gastroesophageal reflux, discussed above, under "Abdominal Pain," in which acid from the stomach regurgitates upwards into the chest area. This is less common in children, but does occur, and often causes a burning pain in the center of the chest.

Don't feel you have to figure out chest pain on your own. A visit to the physician will often sort out whether a significant problem exists. Recognize that most causes are minor and improve with time. However, any chest pain that is severe and persistent, or that causes shortness of breath, needs medical assessment.

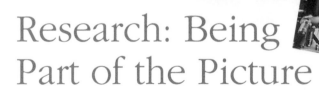

CHAPTER 17

Research: Being
Part of the Picture

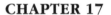

The advice in this book is based not just on the opinions of experienced physicians but on scientific research into what can be *proved* to benefit children with various problems. Because we consider careful medical and clinical research to be of great importance, we want to conclude with a few comments about what research is, and what it means to our children. This is especially important as you and your child may someday be asked to participate in a research project.

Q What's the difference between medical research and clinical research?

Research in the field of medicine includes a variety of approaches to collecting information. It can roughly be divided into *basic medical research* and *clinical research*. Basic medical research usually goes on in specialized laboratories, and involves attempts at understanding the underlying principles of health, diseases, and/or therapies. Patients are rarely involved in this form of research. In contrast, clinical research often involves the participation of patients, and its direct aim is to develop and test better ways of diagnosing and treating people.

Q What happens to patients in a research study?

In many cases, clinical research is limited to measuring or observing the course of health or illness at a given time, or over a time period. Observation may include questions (about illness symptoms, activities, past illnesses, and so on), physical measurements (such as weight and height), and/or tests (such as blood tests or X rays).

Unfortunately, studies like these often fail to reveal whether treatments or tests actually benefit people in a significant way. For this reason another type of clinical study, called a "randomized controlled trial," is sometimes used. This is designed to compare two or more different approaches to treatment. Usually each of the approaches must be either an established treatment, or a new method that is believed to be as good as, or better than, the standard approach. For example, if the usual approach to an illness is to observe it without treatment, and a new drug becomes available to treat the illness, the trial might consist of one group getting observation and another getting the new drug. Both groups would then be evaluated to determine which fared better, and the most successful approach would then become standard.

 Why are these trials called "randomized" and "controlled"?
The groups to be compared have to be similar at the start of the trial (e.g., they should have the same range of severity of illness and be the same mix of ages). Otherwise it may not be clear whether a difference at the end is due to the treatment approach, or to the original differences between the groups. To assure that the groups start out as identical as possible, participants are assigned to the groups by a process of chance called "randomization." This is similar in effect to flipping a coin—if heads are up, the person joins one group; if tails are up, it's the other group—and means that each participant has exactly the same chance of ending up in one group or the other.

The trials are often "controlled" in other important ways. Often the participating patients don't know what treatment they're receiving. In the example above, the group getting the medication might "feel better" just because they *believed* the pills were helping; to keep the test fair, the group not getting medication might be given a placebo (dummy drug) so that they received the same imaginary benefit. Sometimes even the researchers don't know who's getting what, to be sure that their opinions don't affect the results; these are called "double-blind" trials.

Are these studies done on children too?
Clinical research, and in particular randomized controlled trials, play a very special role in improving the medical care of our children. Physicians have learned that even the most thoughtful judgments or expert opinions about how to treat an illness often have to be revised when good studies are finally performed. Also, the illnesses that affect children, and their responses to treatment, are so specific to children that experiments or studies carried out on animals or adults with similar illnesses usually don't tell us how the treatment will affect a child. If we didn't do clinical research with children as participants, we would

be neglecting them. While progress was made in treating adult illness, many of the essential questions about childhood medical care would go unanswered.

Good clinical studies sometimes have a lot of rules for deciding which group a child is placed in, and who can know which treatment a child is receiving, and so on. These rules may seem restrictive, and even frustrating, to parents, but they are usually essential to make the trial reliable. Without them, the validity of the information gained in the study would be in question.

Who runs these clinical studies?

Some physicians are involved in designing and running clinical trials in their hospital departments or practices. Physicians in private practice often play a critical role in referring patients to studies that need to recruit wide participation, and they may play a further role by following the people in the study, gathering information, and helping to ensure that patients get the tests and treatments needed. Note that if a child's physician refers a child to a study, he or she usually *remains* the child's regular physician, with the responsibility of caring for the child's health whether the child remains in the study or not.

If my child takes part in a study, will our doctor necessarily be involved too?

The physician may have very little to do with the research your child participates in. However, even if your child joined the study through another physician or nurse, your child's usual physician will probably appreciate hearing about it. He or she may have advice or support to offer both you and your child. No one has studied whether physicians involved in conducting research, or in referring participants to research studies, provide better care than other doctors. Many of the latter may have an interest in research but not be in a position to participate, or may not have been approached. However, physicians who actively participate may be showing a greater appreciation of the importance of research, and a greater sensitivity to the steady progress of medical knowledge and care. If you have questions about the role your child's physician will play when your child takes part in research, it may be well worth your while to ask him or her about it.

What do I need to understand about my child taking part in research?

Most people recognize that participation should be voluntary, and that participants should understand the purpose and nature of the research they take part in. This means that no one should be forced to join a clinical study through threats, bribery, or fear of not getting treatment otherwise.

As you can imagine, these principles are less easily applied to children. Many simply can't understand the purpose and nature of the research, because they are too young or, in some cases, because of handicaps. They are therefore unable to give meaningful consent.

If people who are incapable of understanding the research are simply left out of clinical studies, the studies will not be complete; also these individuals will be denied the chance to contribute to, or perhaps even benefit from, the research. Therefore, a compromise appears to be the best solution; the parent or guardian examines the purpose and nature of the research, as well as its risks and benefits; makes the decision; and gives permission on behalf of the child if participation seems worthwhile.

Children over seven or eight years of age may be interested in participating in this decision, even if they aren't mature enough to fully understand or appreciate the study. Therefore, their opinion should be considered in addition to that of the parent or guardian. This way, children can participate in and benefit from research, but their rights as individuals are still respected.

How do I find out the purpose and nature of the study?

The physician, nurse, or research assistant who contacts you should be able to outline the key information. In addition, most studies are required to give you a letter explaining the most important aspects. When you receive it, you should be able to see clearly what question the study is designed to answer, and get a sense of whether you feel the study is worthwhile. You should also get a clear description of what the study involves. This includes how long it will run, what tests and treatments will be used (and what these tests and treatments are like), whether your child will be assigned to a particular group and treatment by randomization, and what the alternatives to participation are. You should also be informed of your right to withdraw your child from the study at any time, for any reason.

How do I balance the possible risks and benefits?

When reviewing the study information, pay special attention to the possible risks or harms as well as the benefits. An example of a very minor harm is the discomfort and bruising that occurs when a blood sample is taken from a child's vein. A more significant risk or harm might be the chance of a severe skin reaction to one of the medications being studied, if that medication is known to cause such a reaction.

201

Most treatment approaches, new and old, involve some degree of risk or harm. There are no easy rules for balancing these against the benefits. Yet it makes sense that, for the individual, the potential benefits should outweigh the potential harms. For example, it may be acceptable for a child to have a single blood test for research that will help other children. However, in most cases it's not acceptable to subject a child to many blood tests, or more distressing tests, for research that benefits only other children. In addition to this, the potential risks and benefits of the different approaches in a randomized controlled trial should be fairly balanced. For example, if a new medication is known to have side-effects much worse than those of the traditional medication, and if the potential benefits from the new medication are clearly small, one could argue that the treatments aren't balanced and that the study is improper.

As for the benefits, they can be divided into three categories. First, the study results may help children as a whole, or a specific group of children, through improved medical knowledge. This knowledge may not necessarily benefit your child directly, but your child gains indirectly by helping others, taking pride in this contribution, and knowing that other children continue to contribute in this way. After all, the knowledge from similar studies may have helped your child in the past, or may help in the future. Second, your child may benefit personally from the knowledge gained through the study, if, for example, it compares two medications and clearly indicates which is best. Third, your child may benefit by receiving treatment that is still being tested and is not yet generally available. The extra attention (information, observation, and so on) the child receives may also be beneficial.

Fortunately, you aren't left to balance these issues alone. When a research study is paid for by a large governmental research-funding organization (such as the Medical Research Council or National Health Research Development Program), or by a large charitable foundation (such as the Hospital for Sick Children Foundation), it has already gone through independent, rigorous, competitive review. This review process works towards ensuring that only the best, most scientifically sound studies are selected for funding. These large organizations also require that the studies be reviewed by a special group called an "ethics review board." Ethics review boards are usually made up of people from a variety of backgrounds, such as philosophy, medicine, and nursing, and often include members from the community (at a children's hospital, parents of children who have required medical care are often selected). These groups examine the clinical studies to be sure that the risks and benefits are reasonable, and that appropriate information is given to the parents.

What if the trial is paid for by somebody else?

When clinical studies are paid for by other organizations, such as drug companies, they may not go through quite the same process of review. Most universities and hospitals require all studies conducted on their premises, including those funded by drug companies, to be approved by the ethics review board. However, in some circumstances studies carried out in private offices or clinics may not have undergone ethical or scientific review by an independent group. Because some studies undergo extensive review and others don't, you should feel free to ask who is paying for the study, and what reviews have been done.

Even though these reviews ensure that most clinical studies are appropriate for children to participate in, you and your child have the final decision. Your child's physician may assist you with this, but ultimately you yourself should be satisfied that you understand the benefits and the drawbacks of any research in which your child takes part.

CHAPTER 18

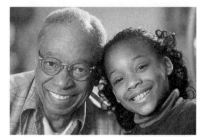

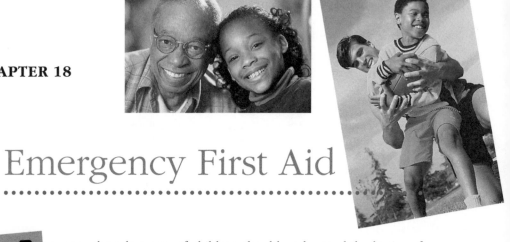

Emergency First Aid

A nyone who takes care of children should understand the basics of first aid. Injuries can happen any time, and the first few minutes can be critical. Even when an injury isn't serious, prompt and appropriate first aid can make the difference between a minor incident, quickly forgotten, and a frightening and upsetting one.

This chapter gives a brief overview of what to do in a few basic emergencies; for more complete and extensive training, take a first-aid course from an agency such as the Red Cross. Even if you never have to deal with a serious situation, the training will change the way you handle day-to-day injuries and mishaps.

Emergency Index

What's involved in taking first aid?

A comprehensive course generally takes either a weekend or four or five week nights. Some teaching is done with books, videos, and/or lectures, but you also spend time trying out practical skills; this can be a lot of fun, especially if you take along a buddy to be your partner. A typical course covers the immediately life-threatening problems of choking, stopped breathing, and severe bleeding, and other topics such as burns, poisonings, cuts, broken bones, sprains, head injuries, and allergic shock. Some courses include CPR (cardiopulmonary resuscitation), but CPR is also taught separately.

Isn't first aid mostly common sense?

While a lot of first aid seems like "common sense" once you've learned it, untrained people can make serious mistakes because they don't understand

Cardiopulmonary resuscitation (CPR)

CPR is a simple technique for helping someone whose heart has stopped beating ("cardiac arrest"). It involves alternately "pumping" the heart by pressing down on the chest, and giving mouth-to-mouth breathing. Although people often associate CPR with heart attacks, the most common situation in which it is used on children is respiratory arrest; that is, the child stops breathing and the heart soon stops beating as a result. A child may stop breathing for many reasons, including:

- choking
- asphyxiation (such as strangling, smoke inhalation, or getting a plastic bag caught over the face)
- near-drowning
- electric shock
- allergic shock (including food allergies and insect stings)
- poisoning (including drug or alcohol overdose)
- an epileptic convulsion
- a diabetic emergency
- a violent blow to the chest (in a fall or collision, for example)

CPR courses generally include first aid for choking and for stopped breathing, since the three conditions often go together. Techniques are slightly different for infants, children aged one to eight, and "adults" over age eight; be sure the course you sign up for includes the age group you are most concerned about.

what's going on in the injured person, or what the first-aid priorities are. Sometimes what seems like the obvious first step is in fact very dangerous.

Besides, it's not easy to stop and think sensibly in an emergency. A good first-aid course does more than just teach you facts; it also drills you in a simple "A B C" routine to help you handle a frightening situation in an organized, logical way. It should give you the confidence to stay calm yourself; to reassure the child; and to *take charge of the scene*, stopping other people from doing damage to the child.

Choking (Any Age)

If the baby or child can breathe or talk or cough, be reassuring but don't interfere; he or she will probably manage to cough up the obstruction. If you do an emergency maneuver on a child who doesn't really need it, you may do unnecessary damage.

If the baby or child can't breathe or talk or cough, or makes only a faint wheezing or whistling sound, follow the steps below. Note that if this isn't your own child, you must have the permission of whoever is in charge of the child. If no such person is present, you don't need permission unless the child is old enough to understand the risk and give "informed consent." After

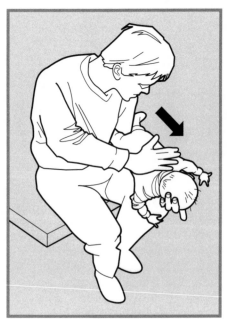

the obstruction is cleared, the child *must be checked by a doctor*, even if he or she seems fine; there is a slight chance that the life-saving maneuver may have caused internal bleeding.

Conscious Choking Baby (under Age One)

If anyone else is around, explain that the baby is choking and ask that an ambulance be called.

Lay the baby face down on your forearm, cradling the face in your hand and pinning one leg between your arm and body. Tilt the baby slightly *head downward* so that gravity will help move the obstruction out.

Use the heel of your other hand to give five blows to the baby's shoulder-blade area. Adjust the force of the blows to the baby's size, to drive out the obstruction without doing unnecessary injury.

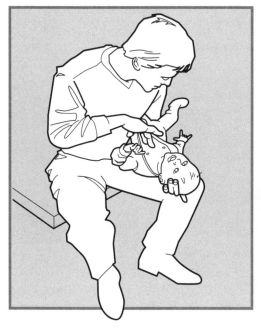 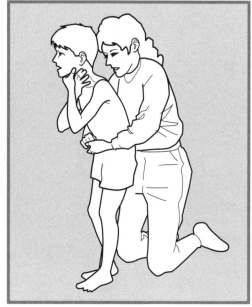

If the choking continues, roll the baby face up on your other forearm, holding the head securely in your hand. Again, tilt the baby slightly head downward. Imagine a line between the baby's nipples; line up your middle three fingers at this line, and then *lift* the top finger and use the other two fingers to thrust straight down five times.

If the choking continues, roll the baby back to the first arm and repeat the maneuvers—five back blows, then five chest thrusts—until the obstruction is clear.

Conscious Choking Child (over Age One)

Stand or kneel behind the child, depending on the child's height. Make one hand into flat-sided fist, thumb outside. Place this fist just above the child's belly-button and cup your other hand over it (see diagram on page 208).

Now pull both hands upward and inward to imitate a forceful "cough." (The larger the child, the harder the motion should be.) If the first few thrusts don't clear the obstruction, continue the maneuver, making the thrusts harder. This is known as the "Heimlich maneuver."

207

The Heimlich maneuver

When we start to choke on something, we usually cough and clear the obstruction out of the way. We need help only if the blockage is so complete that we can't cough hard enough to get rid of it.

For the Heimlich maneuver to be most effective, the flat of the rescuer's fist should be between the victim's rib cage and navel, and each thrust should be as sudden and forceful as a cough. The sudden pressure forces air out of the lungs and, with luck, drives the obstruction out of the airway.

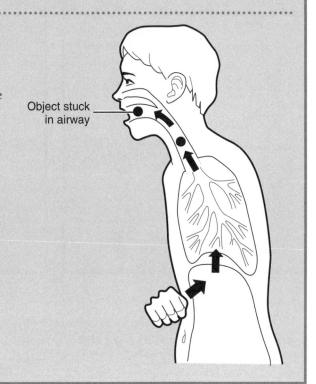

Object stuck in airway

Unconscious (Any Age)

If you can't awaken your child by pinching the earlobes, tapping the soles of the feet, and calling loudly in both ears, the child is likely unconscious. *Call an ambulance at once.*

Unless you suspect a head or spinal injury (see below), gently roll the child onto his or her back, tilt the head up slightly, and see if you can hear or feel breathing, or see the chest moving. If not, call the ambulance dispatcher again and report this as well. Gently roll the child face down on a flat surface, with the head turned to one side and the chin tilted slightly up; this will help keep the throat open and clear so the child can breathe.

If you do suspect a head or spinal injury, check the breathing as well as you can *without moving the child.* As long as the child is breathing, he or she should not be moved except by trained personnel.

Severe Bleeding

Apply pressure to the wound immediately, to stop the bleeding. Use your bare hand, or the child's bare hand, if necessary. It's essential to stop the loss of blood as quickly as possible.

Once you have pressure on the wound, elevate the injured part above heart level, if that's practical and if the child's injuries permit. For example, if the child's foot is bleeding, lay the child down and prop the leg up on pillows. (A child who may have an injury to the neck or back should not be moved.)

Keep the child still, and be reassuring.

For bleeding think RED

R = *rest* (to slow the pulse rate, which in turn slows the bleeding)
E = *elevation* (raising the wound above heart level slows the bleeding)
D = *direct pressure* (to stop the bleeding as quickly as possible)

Find the cleanest dressing you can, and bandage the wound tightly enough to keep pressure on it, but not so tightly that you cut off circulation. *Do not* remove dressings, even if they get soaked with blood; just put new bandages over top. *Do not* remove anything embedded in a cut, but be very careful not to bump the embedded object or to put pressure on it. Seek medical help at once.

Protecting yourself

If you are helping a bleeding child, there is a small chance you may be exposed to blood-borne diseases such as AIDS and hepatitis B. Be sure your first-aid kits have plenty of rubber or latex gloves.

If no gloves are available, you must decide whether to risk the blood contact or not; if you decide to do so, wash thoroughly with soap and hot water as soon after as possible.

Severe Burns

Cool the area immediately; a burn keeps on burning until the skin is cooled down. Applying water is usually the fastest method. The larger the burn is, the less cold the water should be; for example, plunge a burned finger into very cold water; immerse a leg with a large burn in cool water or cover it with a sheet sopped in cool water. Do not use ice water. Remove tight jewelry or clothing before swelling starts, but don't try to remove anything that's stuck to the burn. Do not apply creams or ointments, or any "linty" dressing (such as facial tissue); special jelly-covered burn dressings are available in drugstores.

Burns are more serious in children, and have a high risk of infection. Any significant burn to a child should be checked by a doctor.

Poisoning

If there is an empty package or other evidence of the cause of poisoning, pick it up. *Call a poison control center.* Check the front of your phone book for the number. *Do not* apply home remedies unless you are advised to do so by a poison control center or a doctor.

Where to Find Support and Information

Emergency Numbers

National Health Information Center   1-800-336-4797
People's Medical Society   1-800-624-8773

Useful Addresses

Allergy and Asthma Network
3554 Chain Bridge Road
Suite 200
Fairfax, VA 22030
1-800-878-4403

American Cancer Society
1599 Clifton Road NE
Atlanta, GA 30329
1-800-ACS-2345 [227-2345]

American Heart Association
415 North Charles Street
PO Box 17025
Baltimore, MD 21203
1-800-242-8721

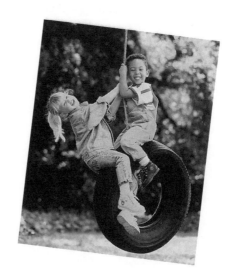

American Lung Association
1740 Broadway
New York, NY 10019
212-315-8700

American Public Health Association
1015 15th Street, NW
Washington, DC 20005-2605
202-789-5661

American Red Cross
17th and D Streets, NW
Washington, DC 20006
202-728-6401

Asthma and Allergy Foundation of America
1717 Massachusetts Avenue, NW
Suite 305
Washington, DC 20036
1-800-7-ASTHMA

Children and Adults with ADD [C.H.A.D.D.]
499 NW 70th Avenue #308
Plantation, FL 33317
305-587-3700

La Leche League International
PO Box 4079
Schaumburg, IL 60168-4079
847-519-7730
Toll free: 1-800-LA LECHE

Learning Disabilities Association of America [LDA]
4156 Library Road
Pittsburgh, PA 15234-1349
412-341-1515

Medic Alert Foundation International
2323 Colorado
Turlock, CA 95381-1009
1-800-ID-ALERT [432-5378]
1-800-344-3226 (for calls within CA)

National Mental Health Association Information Center
1021 Prince Street
Alexandria, VA 22314-2971
1-800-969-6642

Index

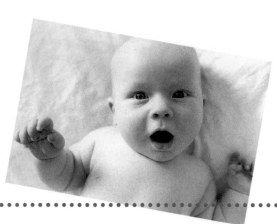

Page numbers in italics denote an illustration.

215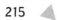